Dear Beck, "knowledge" is power. I believe that the more you understand your diagnosis the more you can deal with it. I hope this book helps (I hope it isn't too graphic.) Good luck in the days to come.

Love,
Donna

Meet Virginia: Biography of a Breast

Jay Agarwal, MD	reconstructive surgeon
Anne Vinsel	photographer
Ravinder Ahluwalia	medical student
Leigh Neumayer, MD MS	mastectomy surgeon

1

2

Table of Contents

A Note about Color

The photographs in this book were taken using natural light, which in surgery is very unnatural indeed. Although everyone involved in the project was very tolerant of the photographer, this tolerance rested on the knowledge that they would never be momentarily blinded by flash lighting, and that large, unsterile lights on stands would not be introduced into their often cramped work spaces.

4

In the OR itself, the surgical field is very brightly illuminated, while the edges of the room are quite dark. This helps surgeons see into body cavities and also helps them concentrate on the area immediately under their gaze, since other areas drop off into darkness. The old term "operating theater" reflects surgical lighting, with bright spotlights and pools of darkness.

The patient's skin is usually swabbed with Betadine, a yellow-brown solution that turns Caucasian skin bright yellow. Lighting in clinics is often quite yellow as well.

All of these considerations can render these surgical photographs somewhat strange in their color balance. I chose to leave them as is, and the photographs are what you would see if you were in the room observing.

Anne Vinsel, photographer

5

Narrative Voices

We used several "voices" in this book. For Part 1, the voice is Dr. Neumayer, the surgeon who performed the mastectomy and for Parts 2 and 3 the voice is Dr. Agarwal, the surgeon who performed the breast reconstruction.

After her surgery, our patient, Shauna, made some comments on an early draft of the book. Her comments are included here in *italics.*

Meet Virginia was created as a collective effort to help educate patients and physicians about breast cancer and reconstruction. Our goal with this book is to highlight the surgical aspects of breast cancer treatment and to enlighten the reader about the possibilities that exist for restoring the female form. Our days consist of consultations with women who are scared, sad, angry and confused about the prospects of life with breast cancer and the deformity that may result. With this book, we hope to educate women about current surgical techniques and to offer them a glimpse of what lies ahead.

By no means is this book comprehensive, nor does it depict what every woman with breast cancer will go through. *Meet Virginia* takes the reader through the treatment and transformation of one woman as she moves forward on this difficult journey.

7

Introduction to Breast Cancer

Breast cancer is a very common disease; nearly 200,000 women are diagnosed in the United States each year. Fortunately, most women survive and go on to live long healthy lives. That is our goal with every patient.

8

Breast cancer can be either invasive or pre-invasive. The pre-invasive type is called Ductal Carcinoma *in situ* (DCIS). This means that the breast cancer cells have not broken through the lining of the ducts. Once this happens, the cancer is categorized as invasive breast cancer.

DCIS is basically a pre-invasive form of breast cancer. If left alone for ten years or so, 50% of the time it will develop into an invasive cancer. Therefore, especially in younger women, we tend to treat it much like an invasive cancer. The biggest difference between the treatment of DCIS and invasive cancer is that we may not sample lymph nodes in a patient with only DCIS. This is because it is highly unlikely that the cancer cells have made it to the lymph nodes, since they haven't made it past the lining of the ducts.

However, it is currently recommended that women who either choose or are recommended to have a mastectomy for DCIS should have a sentinel node biopsy at the time of the mastectomy. The reasoning behind this is that there is always a possibility that there is a small invasive cancer in the breast and if a sentinel node biopsy is not done at the time of the mastectomy, it cannot be done later. If an invasive cancer is found and a sentinel node biopsy was not done, the patient will have to undergo a complete axillary lymph node dissection.

Although many parts of the treatment of pre-invasive and invasive breast cancer are similar, there are some differences. First, we will go over the treatment for invasive breast cancer. The overall treatment of invasive breast cancer is dictated in large part by the characteristics of the tumor. These characteristics are also what predict how good or bad the cancer is or might be. The four basic characteristics are:
1. Size of the tumor
2. Whether or not lymph nodes are involved
3. Grade of the tumor (what the cells look like under the microscope)
4. Whether or not there are hormone receptors (docking stations) on the cancer cell wall

Size of the tumor and lymph node involvement are pretty self explanatory. Grade of the tumor refers to how the cells look under the microscope. There are three grades:

Grade 1--well differentiated-the cells look pretty well behaved

Grade 2--moderately differentiated-the cells are looking a little more crazy/aggressive

Grade 3--poorly differentiated-the cells look aggressive and aren't behaving (aren't forming glands, etc.)

Hormone receptors (estrogen and progesterone receptors) are essentially docking stations on the cell wall for the estrogen and the progesterone in your body. When the hormones dock into these stations, they stimulate the cancer cells to grow and divide. It is a good thing to have positive hormone receptors because we have many drugs to block those or to keep you from making the hormones.

Our patient had a very small invasive ductal cancerous tumor and negative nodes. Therefore she did not need chemotherapy or post mastectomy radiation therapy and she was able to complete her surgical treatment and reconstruction in well under a year. Patients who need chemotherapy will either have it before their mastectomy (neoadjuvant) or after their mastectomy (adjuvant). This lengthens the treatment process and time to complete reconstruction to nearly a year.

Some patients will need radiation treatments after mastectomy. The current indications for this are:

    Inflammatory or locally advanced breast cancer (involving skin)
    Large invasive cancer (bigger than 5 centimeters/1.97 inches)
    Close margins (cancer within a millimeter/.04 inches of where the surgeon cut to remove the breast tissue)
    Positive lymph nodes

In our practice, patients who need post mastectomy radiation treatments usually have a tissue expander placed at the time of the mastectomy. The tissue expander can be expanded a little bigger than they think they might want to be and then we radiate them with the expander still in place. After a few months, they can have their final surgery. Radiation can cause scar tissue, though, and frequently this causes asymmetry (the radiated reconstructed breast is surrounded by more scar tissue, making it seem harder and less mobile).

Total skin sparing mastectomy refers to leaving the entire skin envelope of the breast, including the skin of the nipple and areola. Several different skin incisions can be used for this. We have the least amount of skin loss (where the skin dies because of lack of blood supply) using a radial incision that starts at the outer edge of the areola and extends toward the outer portion of the breast.

11

Skin sparing mastectomy refers to leaving most of the skin envelope but removing the skin of the nipple and areola. This is frequently performed by making an incision all the way around the areola.

Traditional mastectomy refers to removing at least an ellipse (football shape) of skin with the breast. This results in a straight line scar where the nipple used to be.

The decision on which mastectomy to do is based on a couple of things. First, if the tumor has grown through the skin in any place, that skin should be removed. Patients with inflammatory breast cancer should have a traditional mastectomy. Patients who have cancers right under the nipple should probably have that skin removed.

There is one other characteristic of the tumor that helps us determine treatment; the her-2-neu receptor. While having this receptor apparent on the cell wall is a marker of a more aggressive tumor, we now have a drug that targets just those receptors and kills only the cells with those receptors (trastuzimab or herceptin).

These characteristics (tumor size, lymph node involvement, grade and hormone status) help us decide how aggressively to treat you. In general, for women under age 70 who are otherwise healthy, we would recommend chemotherapy in addition to surgery if the tumor is greater than 2 centimeters/.8 inches in size, or if the lymph nodes are involved. For some women (younger women, women with tumors that are hormone receptor negative, and/or high grade) we recommend chemotherapy for tumors that are between 1 and 2 centimeters/.4 and .8 inches. For most patients we can estimate the size of the tumor initially by imaging or palpation, and we often have the grade and hormone status from the initial biopsy. Lymph node status is a bit harder to assess. If we feel an enlarged and/or hard lymph node in your armpit, we will frequently try to confirm whether or not there is tumor in the lymph node by sticking a needle in it and pulling out cells.

Most women, however, don't have enlarged lymph nodes that need to be sampled with a needle. In this situation, at the time of their breast surgery, we perform what's called a sentinel lymph node biopsy. This is a technique that allows the surgeon to identify the first couple of lymph nodes that the breast drains to and remove only those nodes. These "sentinel nodes" are then looked at very closely by the pathologist (often while you are still asleep in the operating room) to see if there are any cancer cells in them. If no cancer is seen, then no more lymph nodes need to be removed. If more than a little bit of cancer is seen, we usually recommend an axillary lymph node dissection. Occasionally, there is only a little bit of cancer in the sentinel nodes. If this is the case, sometimes we don't need to do an axillary lymph node dissection.

The sentinel node technique involves injecting dye (radiolabeled material and/or blue dye) into the breast prior to beginning the operation. The dye is picked up in the lymph channels in the breast and gets hung up in the first couple of lymph nodes the breast drains to. The surgeon then uses a Geiger counter (for radiolabeled dye) and their vision (if blue dye is used) to find those lymph nodes. The nodes that are "hot" and/or "blue" are removed for further evaluation.

If we find cancer cells in the lymph nodes by needle aspiration, we know then that you will definitely be recommended to have chemotherapy and that we will need to perform an axillary lymph node dissection (removing 10-15 of the 60 lymph nodes from under your arm).

Surgery is also used to take care of the breast cancer in the breast. For most women, there are three options from which to choose for the local treatment of the breast.
These are:
    Lumpectomy alone
    Lumpectomy followed by radiation treatments
    Mastectomy

We know from a couple of very large randomized trials that there is no difference in survival amongst these groups. This is because survival is dependent on the characteristics of the tumor, not what we do to the breast.

As you might imagine, the less you do to the breast, the higher the likelihood of cancer coming back in the breast. From the study done in the U.S., wherein women with cancers measuring up to 4 centimeters were allowed to participate, we know that lumpectomy alone is associated with a 30-40% local recurrence rate at 20 years. Adding radiation decreases that rate by half; in other words the local recurrence rate 20 years after lumpectomy and radiation treatments is 15-20%. Turning that figure around, there is an 80-85% chance it WON'T come back in the breast. A mastectomy does not completely remove the risk of local recurrence. You can still have a recurrence on the chest wall or in the skin or in the scar. This rate is about 3-5% at 20 years, and perhaps as high as 7% if the entire skin envelope is saved (total skin sparing mastectomy).

In general the choice of treatment options for the local treatment of the breast lies solely with the patient. My recommendation is that we as surgeons should strive for a reasonably good looking breast in the end. Most people would not be happy with a malformed breast where the nipple is pointing toward the armpit or the floor or one with a large dent in it, but truthfully if there are not anatomic factors pushing toward mastectomy, the person who gets to make the final decision is the patient.

Leigh Neumayer, MD

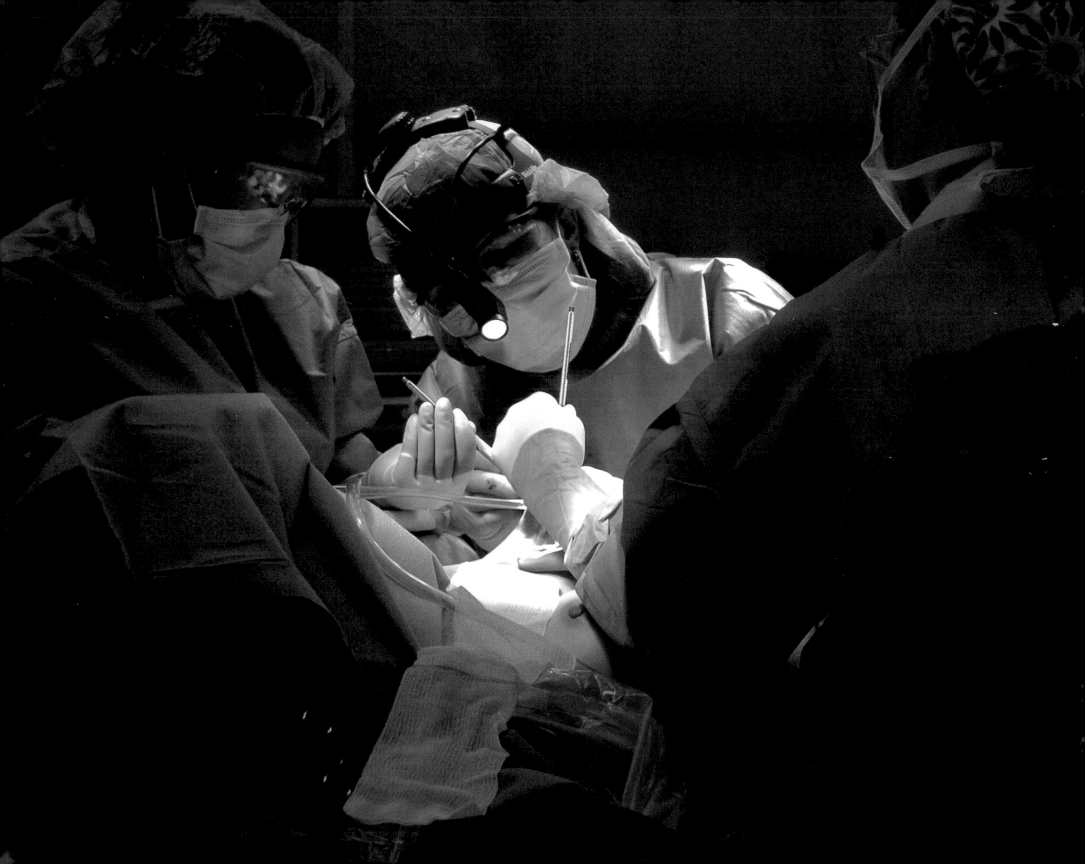

Section 1: Total Skin Sparing Mastectomy

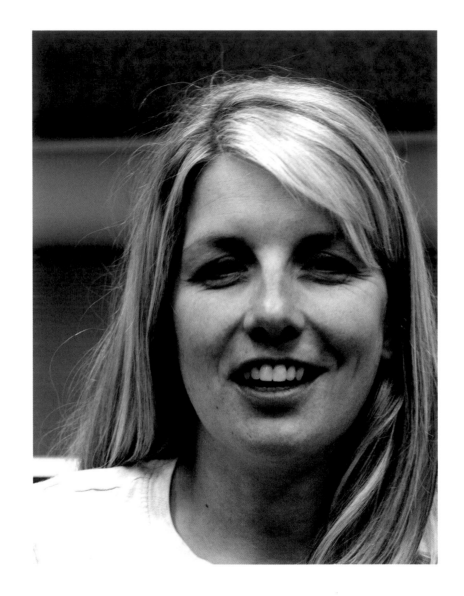

This is Shauna Smith, the patient who allowed us to photograph her during her mastectomy and reconstruction surgeries. Shauna works in rehabilitation and teaches sports to people with severe physical disabilities.

She agreed to participate in this project because she understands the need for information that patients and their physicians can use to communicate with each other about what will happen during surgery.

Shauna inspired the title of this book after we asked her to name the breast that was going to be operated on, so that she and the photographer could discuss the project in waiting rooms or the cafeteria. Shauna settled on "Virginia", because to her that name symbolizes a woman who is quirky and rebellious but also lovable, which is close to the way Shauna feels about the breast with the tumor.

Meet Virginia shows breast cancer surgeries, including a total skin sparing mastectomy and reconstruction with a tissue expander, followed by permanent implant placement. It also shows how we fill the tissue expanders and the subsequent clinic visits to prepare for the final reconstructive surgery. The first two surgeries, the mastectomy and the placement of the tissue expander were performed on the same day by two surgeons, Dr. Neumayer and Dr. Agarwal. Dr. Agarwal also performed the final surgery, the placement of the permanent implant, several weeks after the first OR day, once Shauna's tissue had been gradually stretched to receive the final implant.

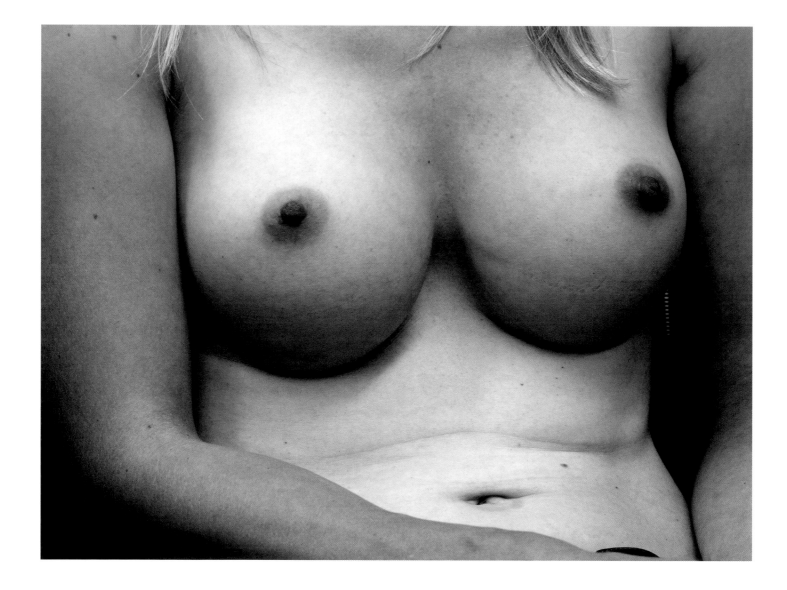

Shauna's breasts before surgery. She previously had breast implants inserted.

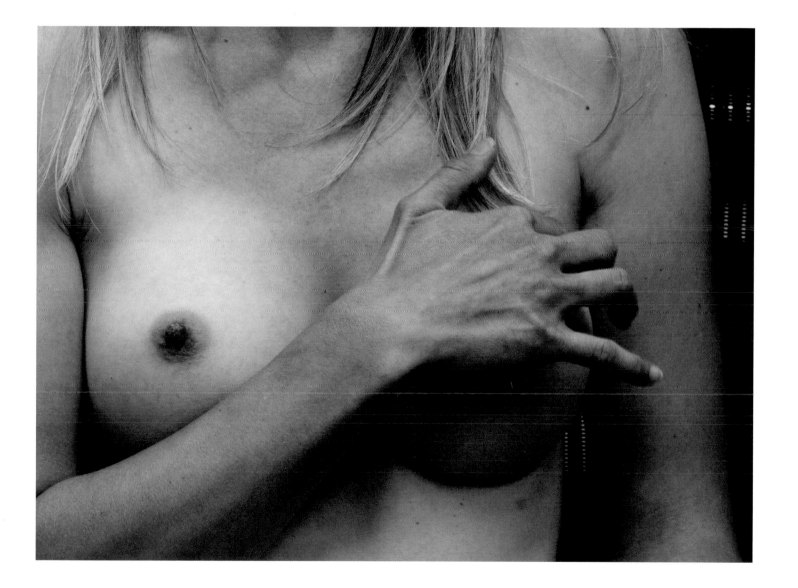

Shauna points to where her tumor is.

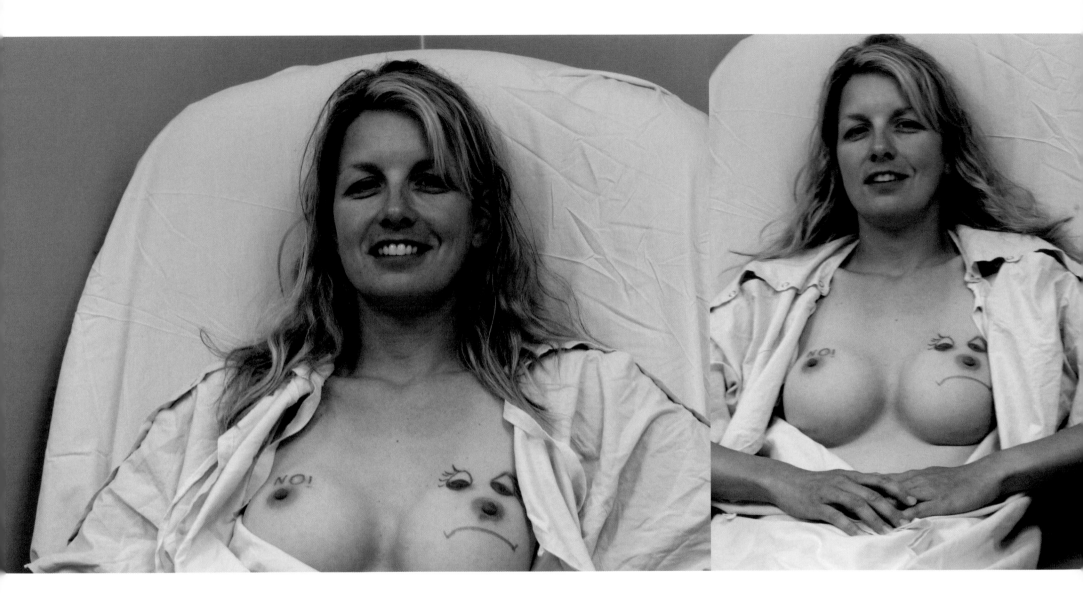

(left) Shauna had to come in early for her mastectomy because she was also going to have a sentinel node biopsy, and the radioactive tracer has to be injected well before surgery.

(right) Shauna's mood varies a little bit from apprehensive to eager to get it over with. She drew on her breasts the night before to lighten the mood.

Throughout this book, Shauna will comment on selected photos. Her "voice" will be in italics:

There were so many people on the scene who assisted me. I frequently felt overwhelmed by how many people had seen me with my shirt off. Just before this surgery I had counted at least 35. I even dismissed an assistant from my first clinic visit from the exam room because I thought he was just another medical student observing. I found out later he had helped with the surgery. I'm grateful for him now. I would say there are 35-60 people who will help you on the path to healing.

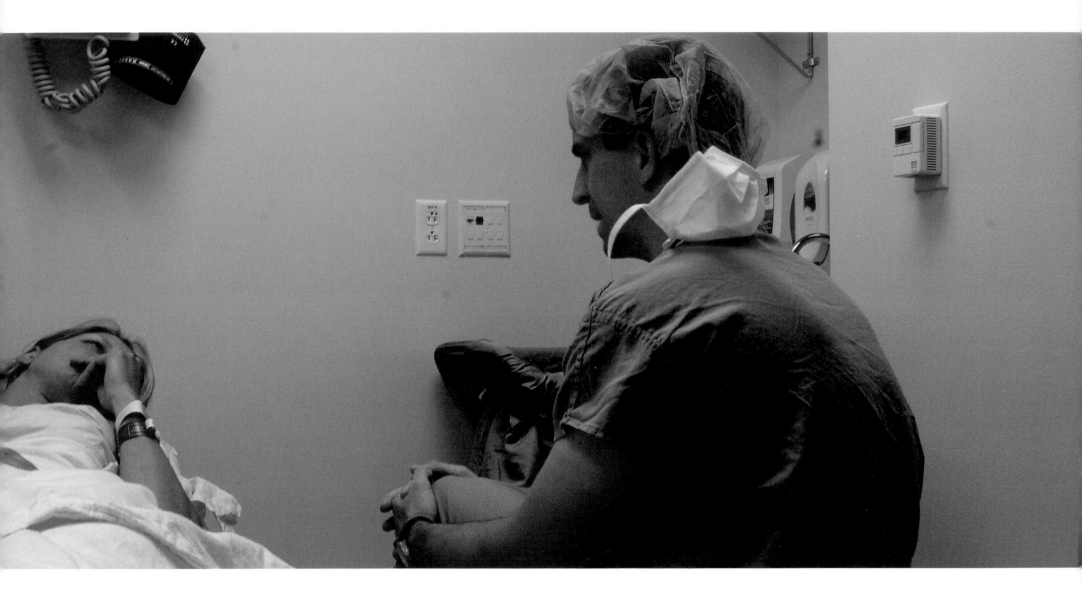

The anesthesiologist visits with Shauna before surgery.

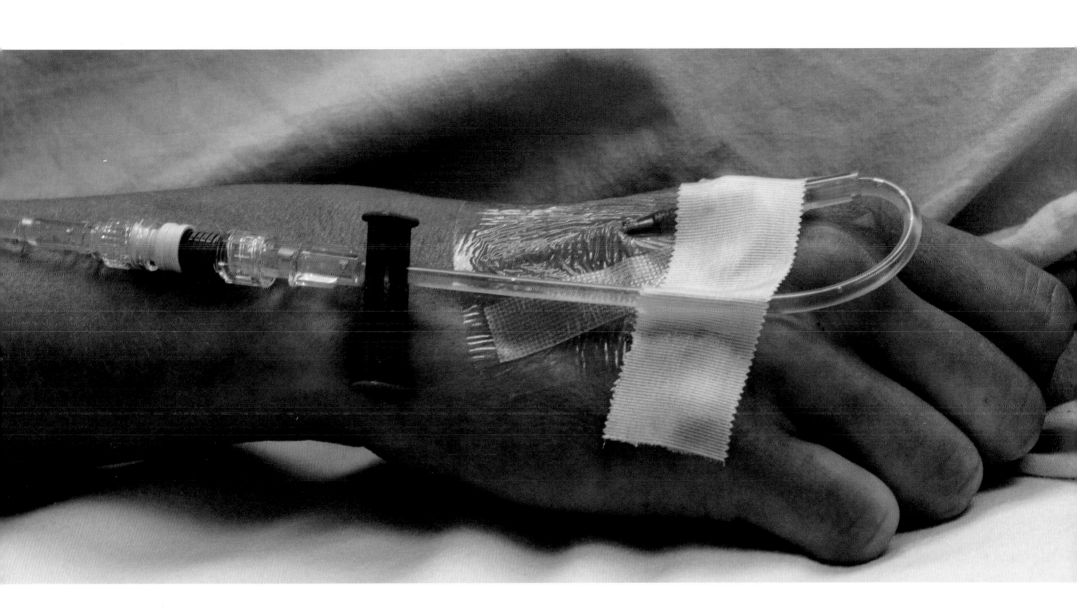

An IV is required for this operation. The anesthesiologist will use it to give Shauna medicines to put her off to sleep.

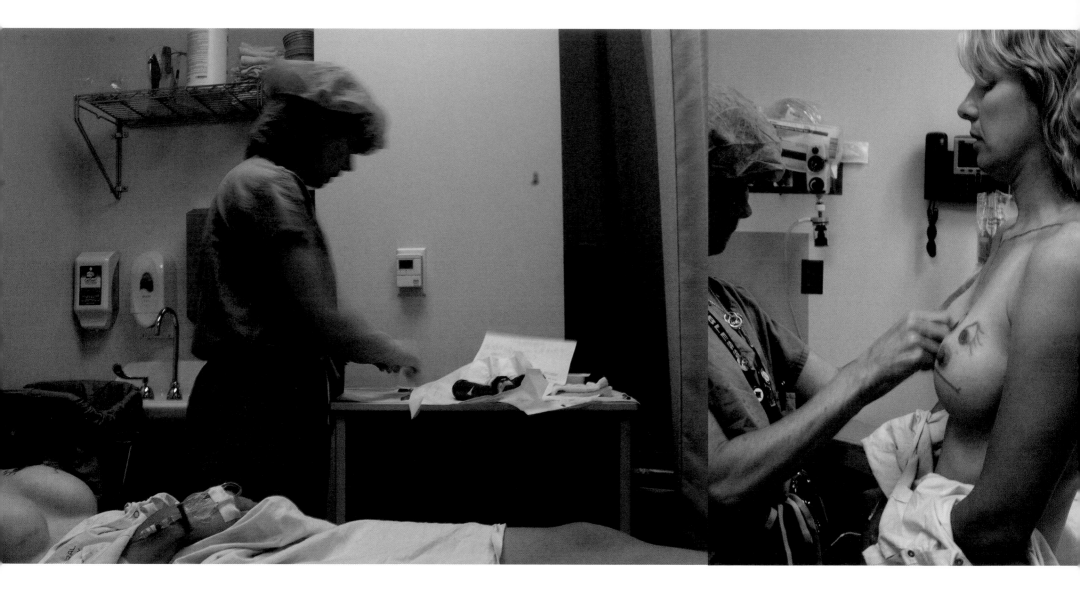

(left) Shauna will be having a sentinel node procedure. We inject dye (radiolabeled) into the breast tissue prior to the patient going to sleep. I use a subareolar technique, wherein I inject 1 cc/.04 oz. containing 1 millicurie into the subareolar breast tissue. I follow this with a 0.05 cc/.002 oz. injection containing 0.2 millicuries in the dermis (skin) of the upper outer quadrant. When we first learned the technique we were taught a "peritumoral" technique that required injecting 8 cc/.32 oz. of the dye into the breast tissue. This was very painful for the patients so I changed to the smaller volume technique. The injections still sting, but not nearly as much.

I use the glove wrapper as a receptacle for all the things that have been in contact with the radiolabeled material. The nuclear medicine department has to follow strict guidelines about disposing of this material. The amount of radioactivity involved in a sentinel node procedure is exceedingly small, but even so it is not approved for use in pregnant women, and I recommend any patient who has had an injection not to hold a child less than one year old to their chest for 24 hours following the injection.

(right) On the day of surgery, we mark the patient. Not only a "yes" on the operative site(s), but for mastectomies I like to mark the landmarks--clavicles (collar bones), middle of the sternum (breastbone) and the inframammary folds (crease under the breast). I do this with the patient standing as everything moves once the patient lies down.

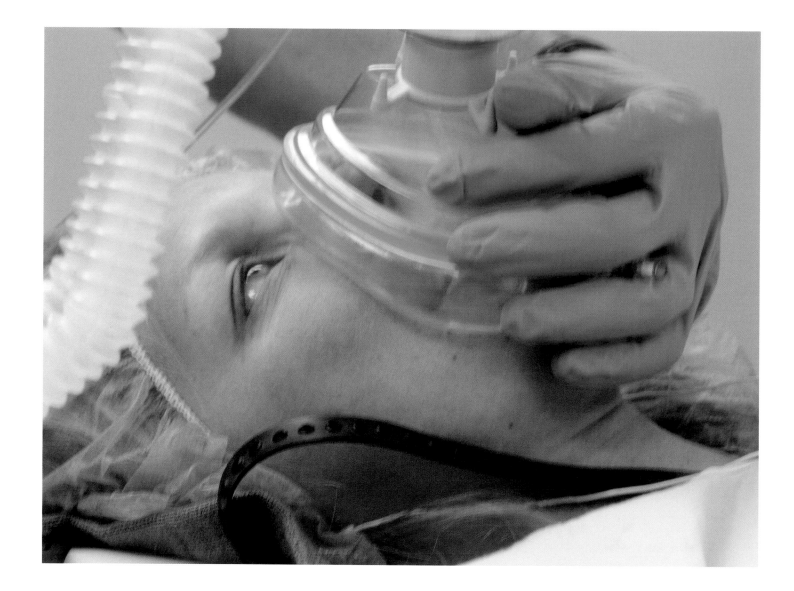

Prior to induction, Shauna is asked to fill her lungs with 100% oxygen. Her heart rate and rhythm, blood pressure and oxygen saturation are also monitored. You can tell Shauna had a "cocktail" of medicines as she is going off to sleep.

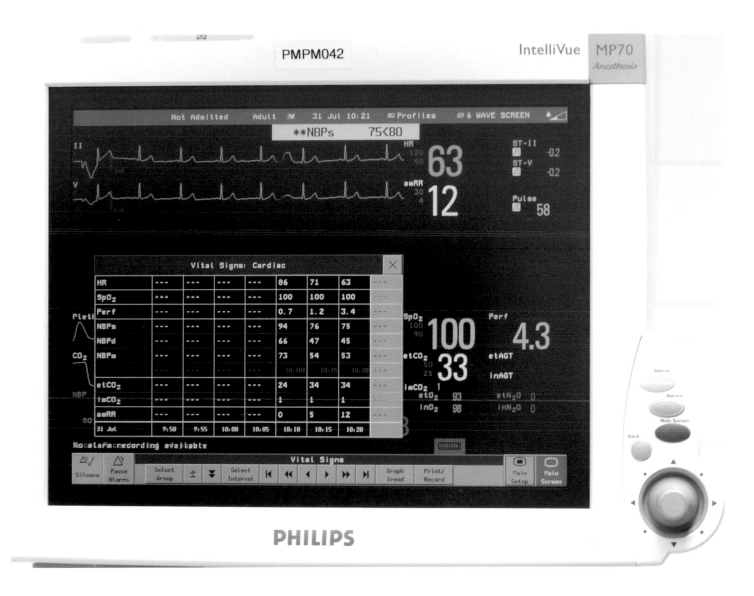

This is the machine that monitors heart rate, respiration rate, oxygen saturation and CO2 (carbon dioxide) breathed out during the surgery.

30

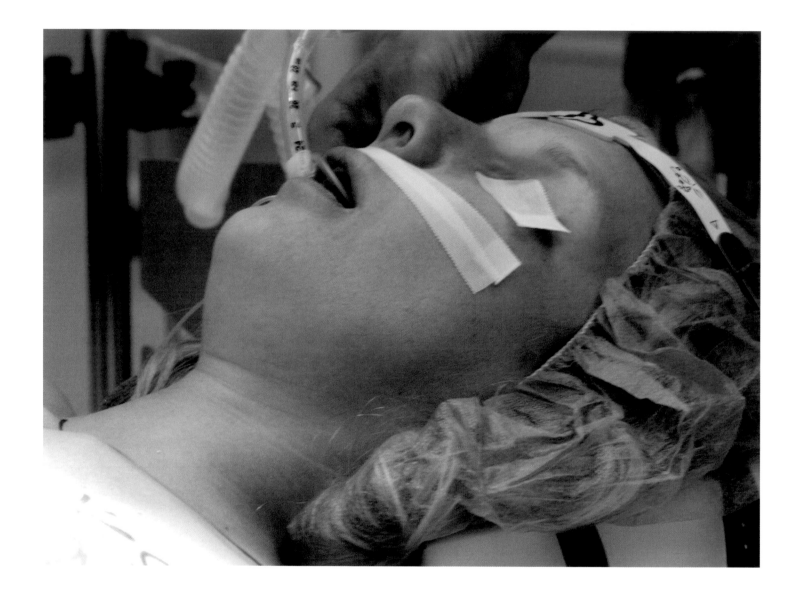

Here is Shauna once the breathing tube is in place. When you are under a general anesthetic, you lose the reflex to close your eyes if something comes close, so Shauna's eyes are lubricated and her eyelids are taped closed.

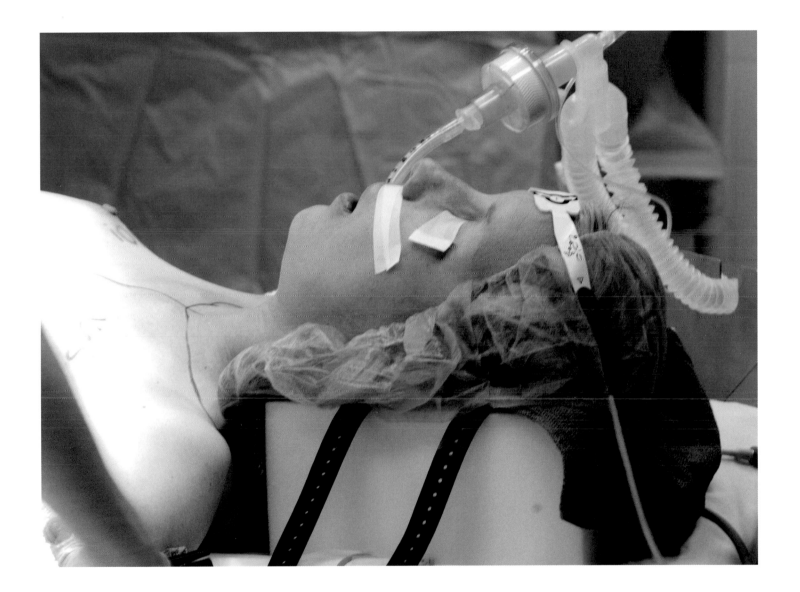

The tape strip on Shauna's forehead is a monitor the anesthesiologists use to help determine how deep Shauna's anesthetic is. Some believe this monitor can prevent people from waking up during their operation.

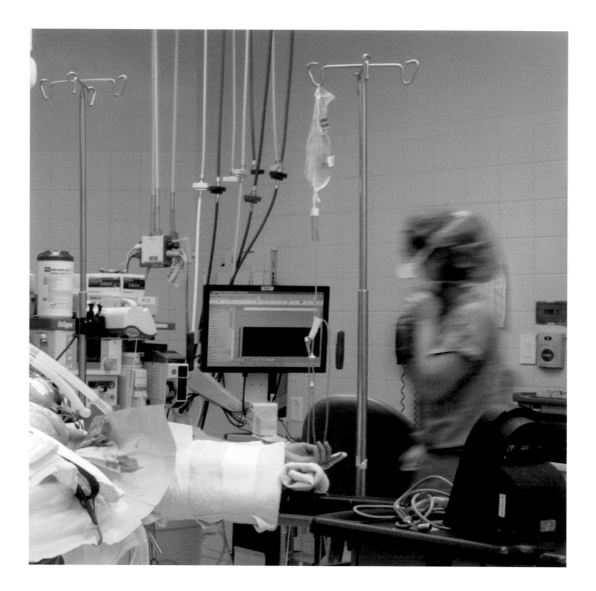

After the patient is asleep, we position her for the operation. I like to pad and secure her arms to the arm boards with towels, so that as we change the position of the table, everything is secure.

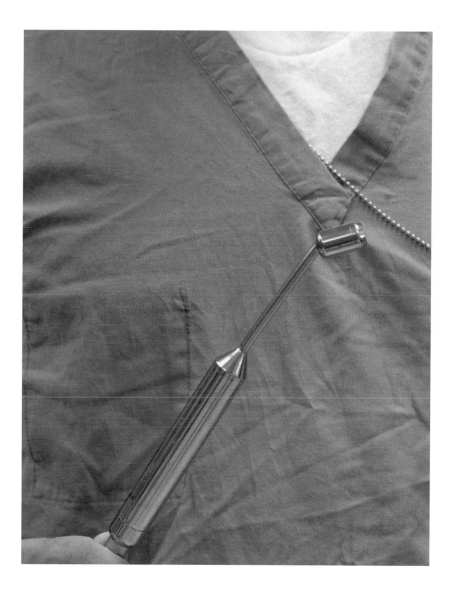

This is the probe part of the Geiger counter.

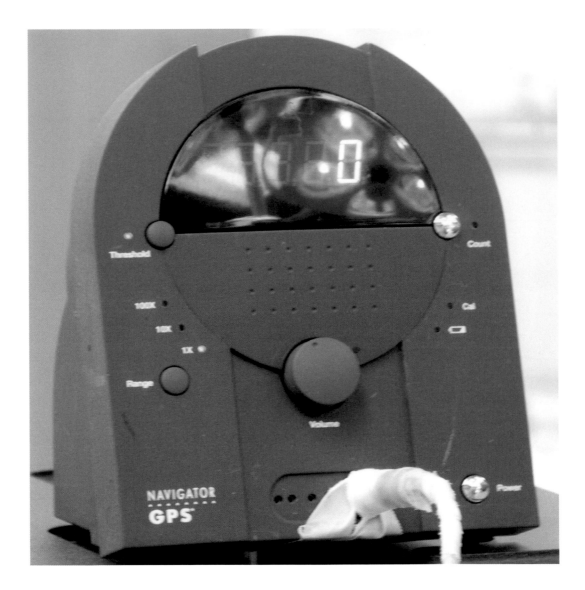

This is the counter part of the Geiger counter. It reminds us of a character in star Wars so we affectionately call it "R2D2."

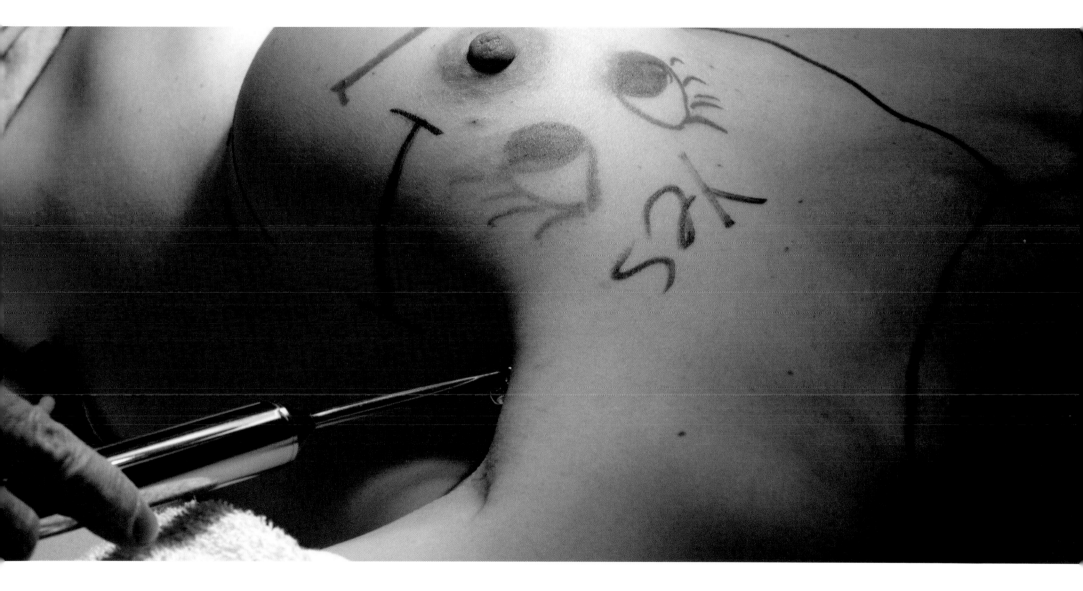

Once the patient is asleep, I use R2D2 to find the "hot spot," an area in the armpit that represents a collection of the radiolabeled dye in a lymph node.

36

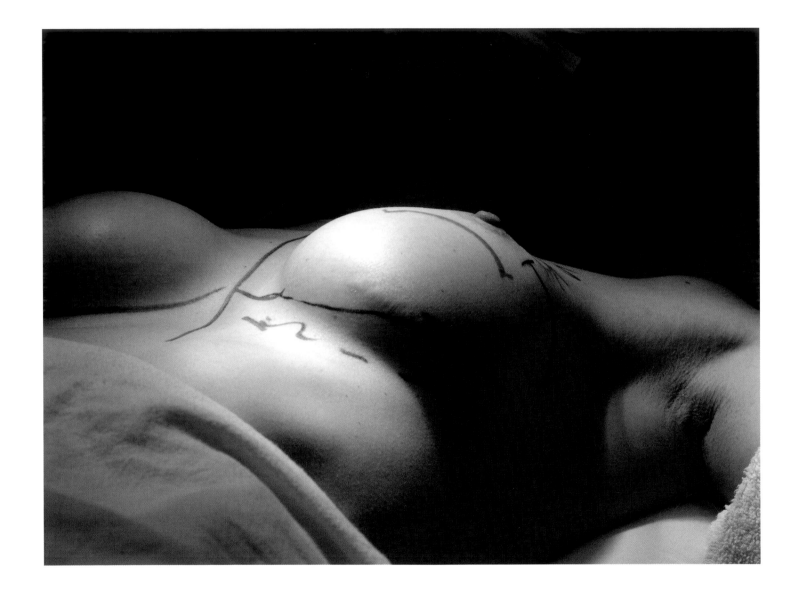

Now we are performing our time out. This is a mandatory step prior to the start of any operation, where we confirm the right patient, right procedure, right (correct) side and that we have everything we need.

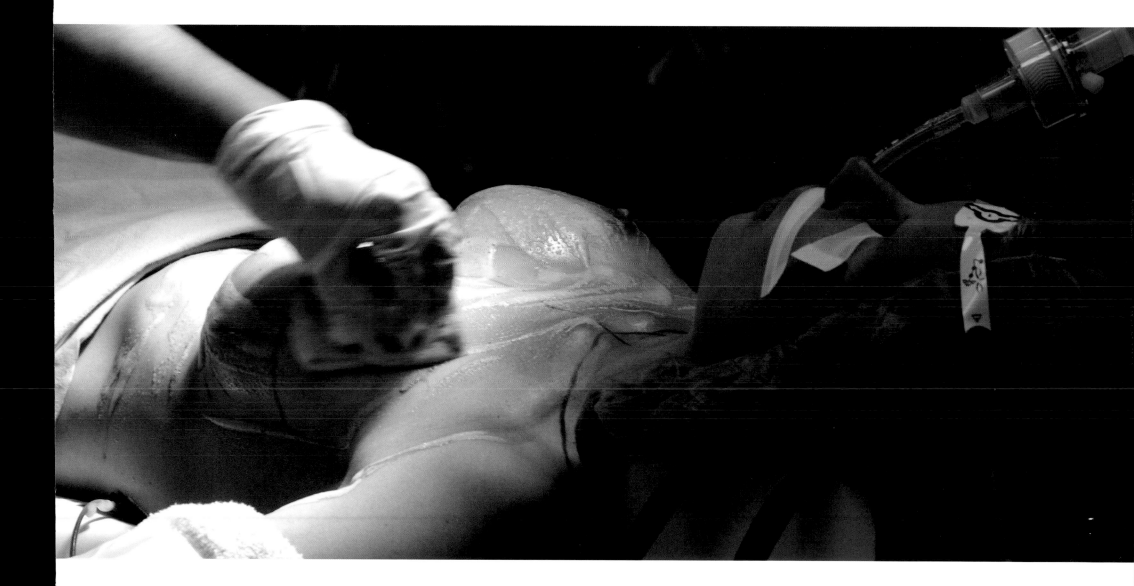

We are prepping (washing) the operative field. Even though we only plan to remove one breast, we have both sides exposed to help with symmetry.

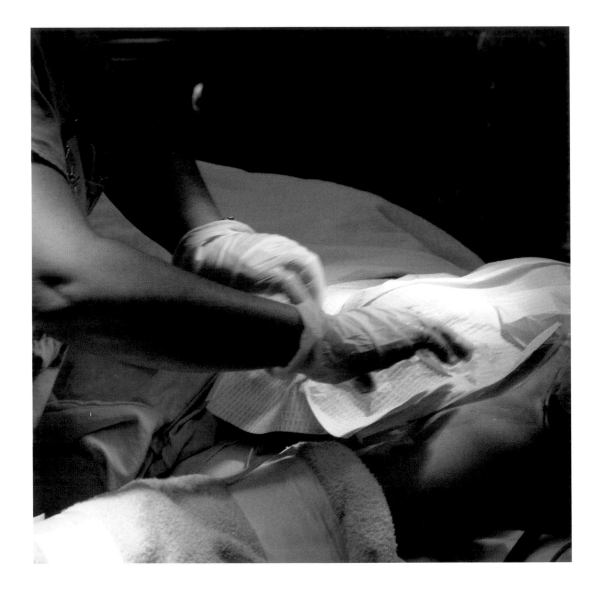

After the prep we dry the field with a sterile towel.

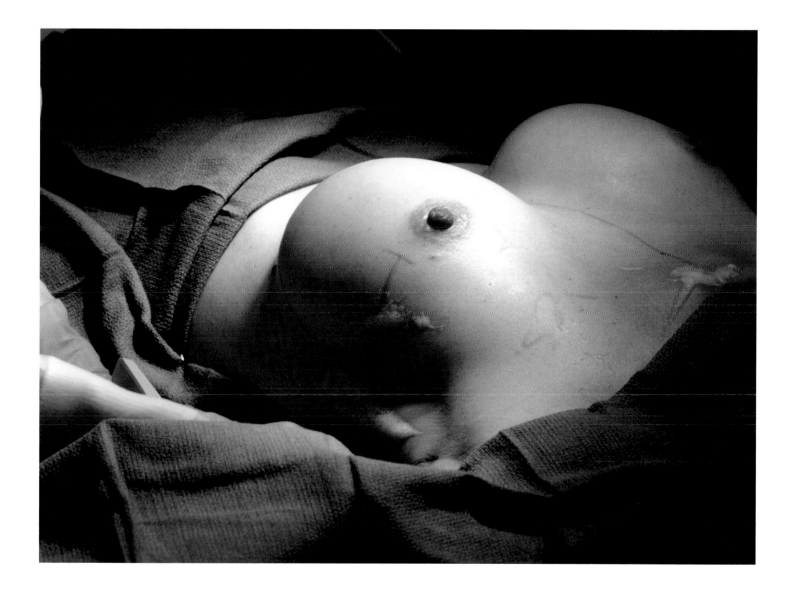

Next we drape with blue towels. As you can see there are lots of nooks and crannies so I use a skin stapler to hold the drapes in place.

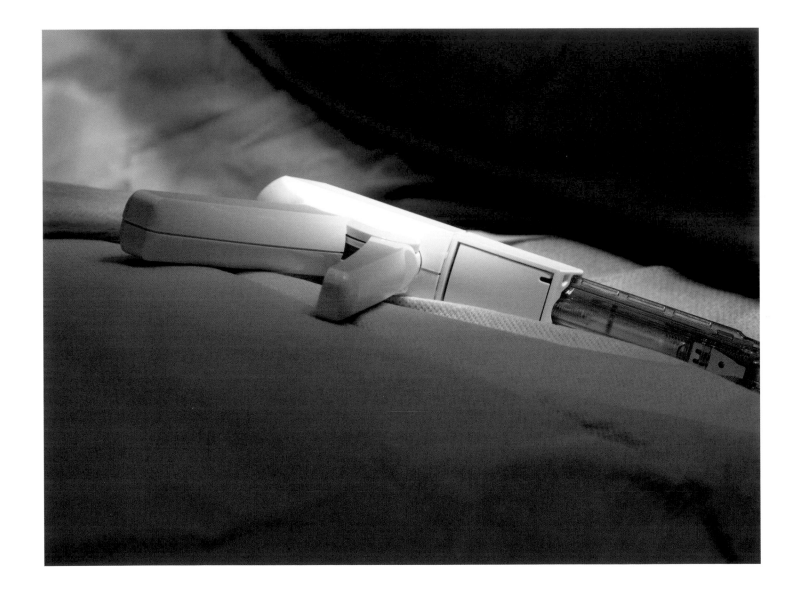

This is the skin stapler. It leaves little marks that disappear in a day or two.

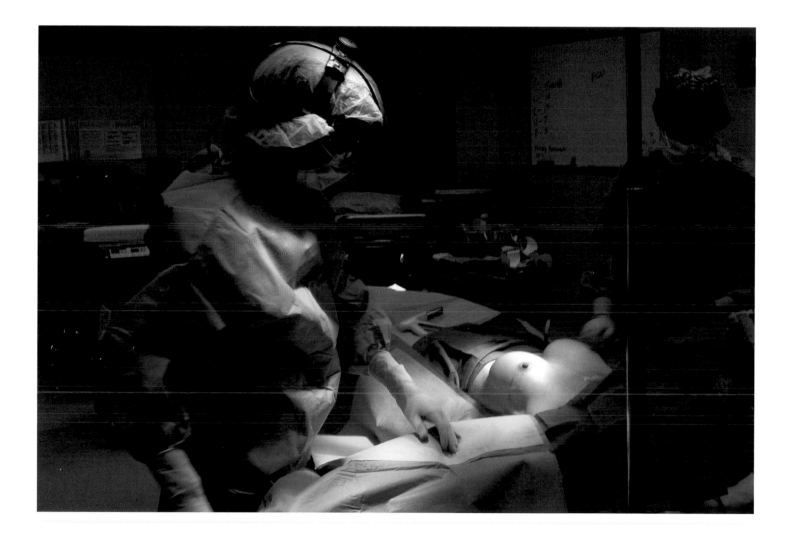

We follow the blue towels with a layer of paper drapes.

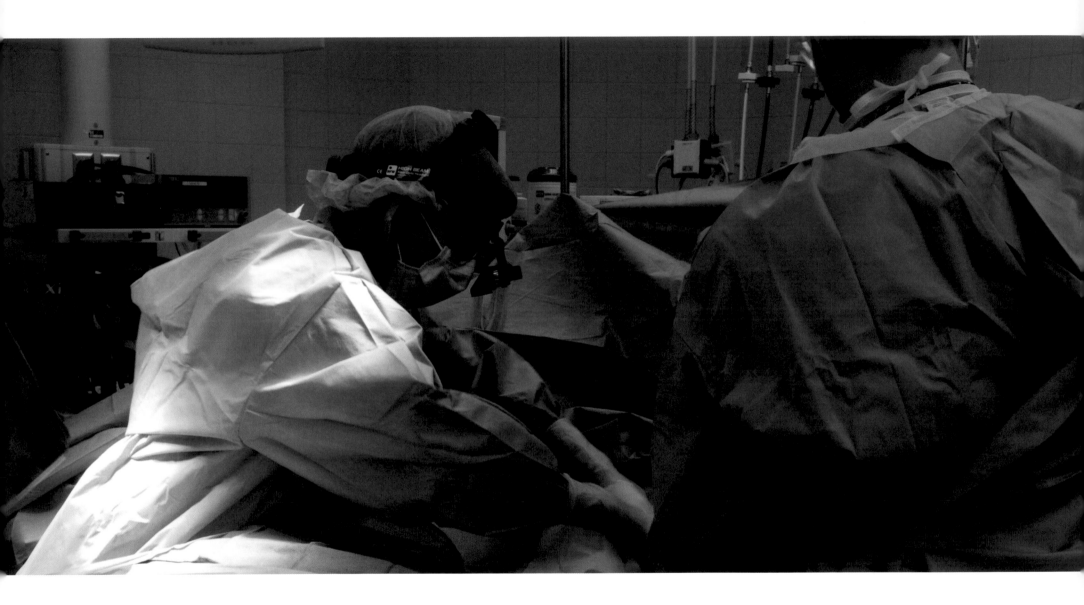

We cover basically everything in order to have a sterile field. Everything in blue is now sterile.

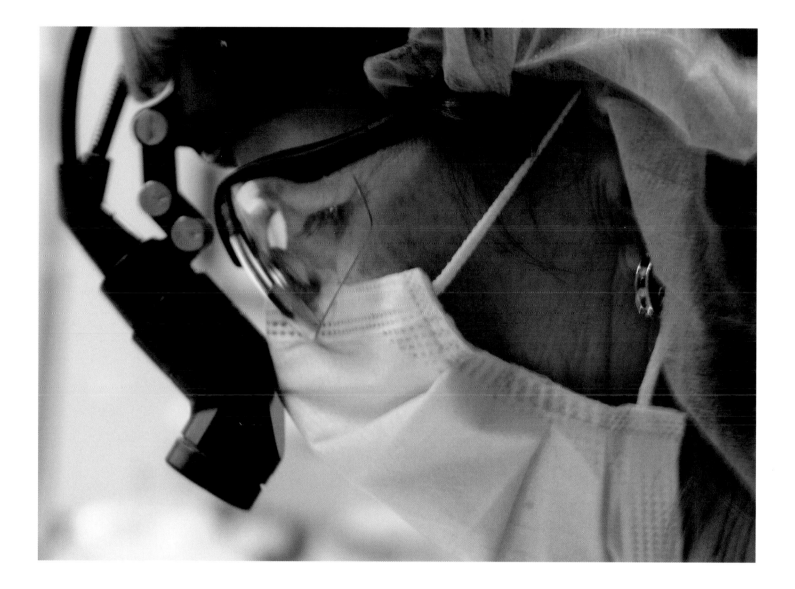

43

Now we can start the surgery. For these procedures I wear a head lamp. I try to keep my incisions as small as possible. The light on my head illuminates exactly where I am looking. I make the incision with a scalpel.

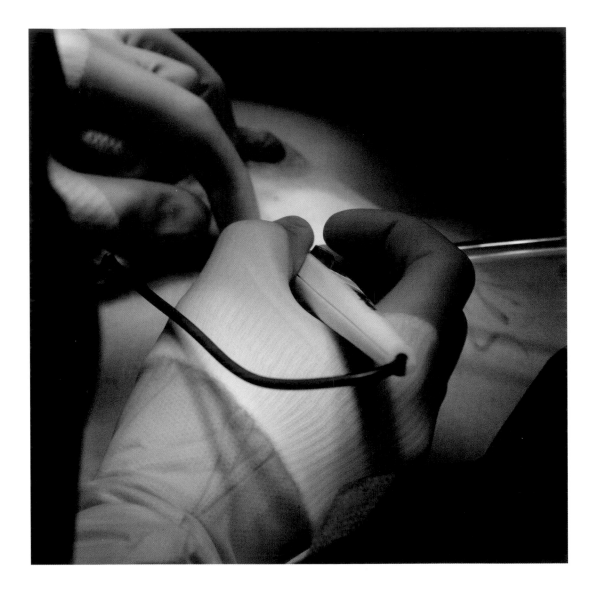

Once I have incised through skin, I use electrocautery to do the dissection.

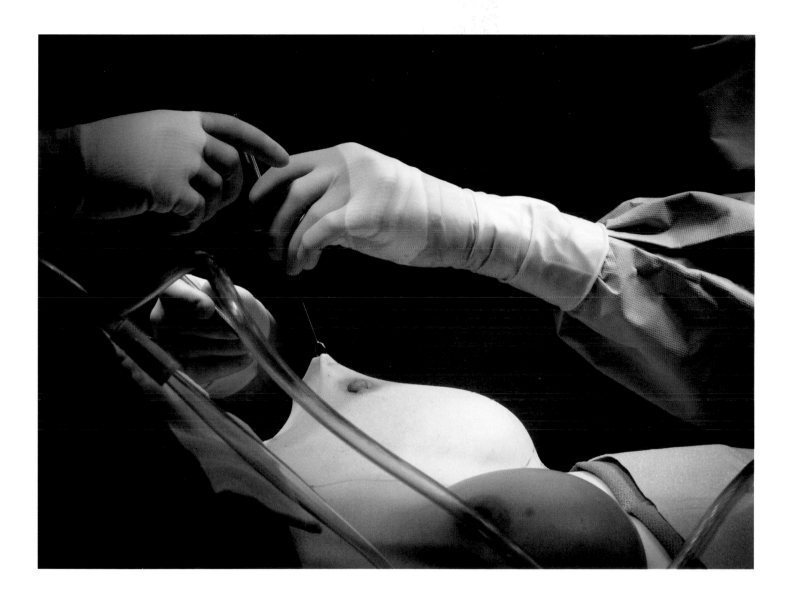

This operation requires good use of traction and counter traction. Here we are placing skin hooks to help elevate the skin flaps. It is important to pull straight up to the ceiling with the hooks.

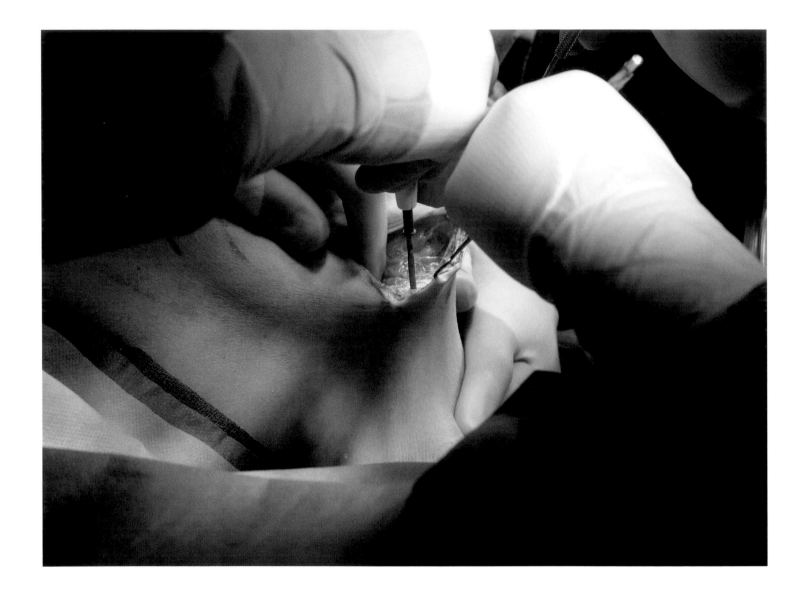

Now, the electrocautery wand is used to dissect between the subcutaneous tissue and the breast tissue.

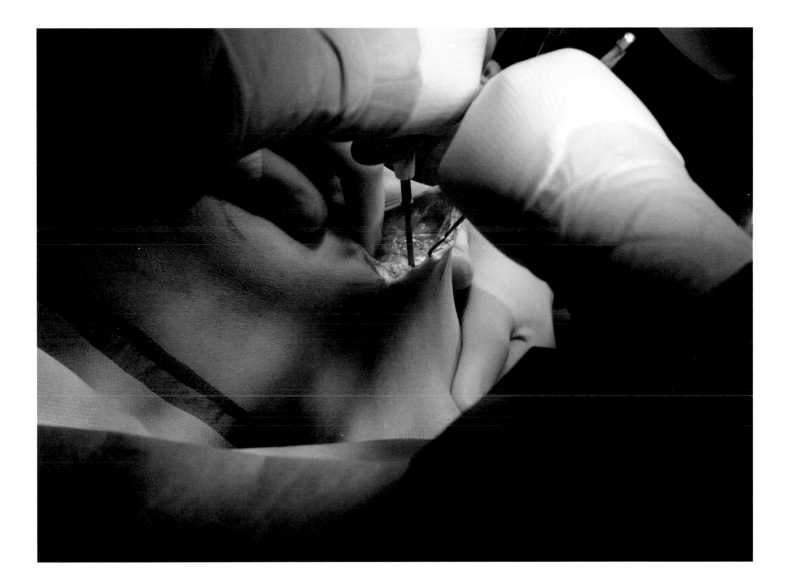

In most women, with the right amount of traction a nice filmy plane is apparent.

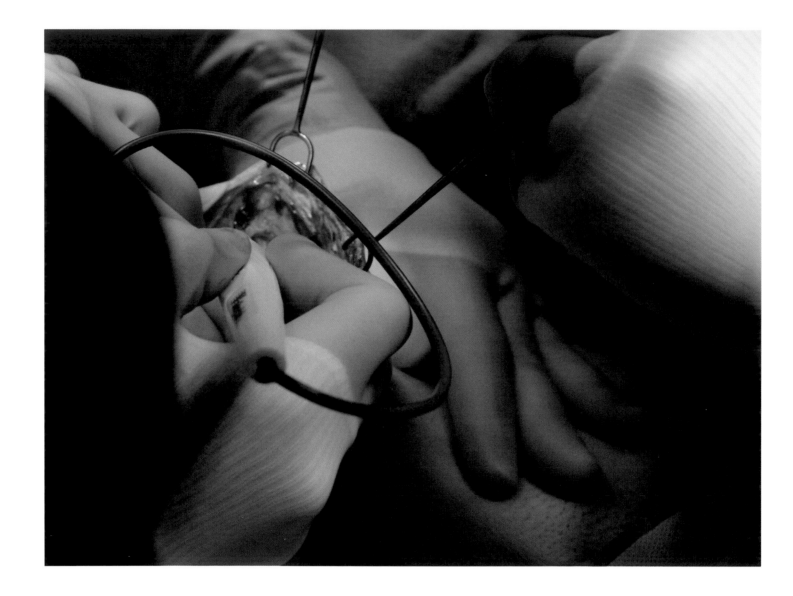

The hole is small. The black spots are where there were vessels that needed to be cauterized. The hand above the incision is providing countertraction. It makes the plane of dissection easier to see.

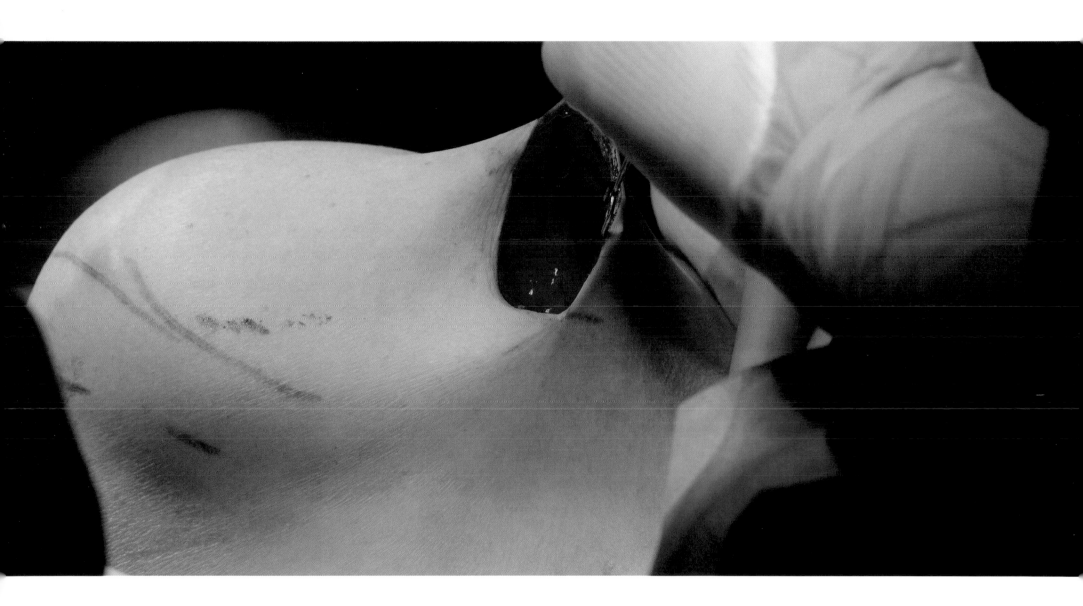

Despite a small incision, by working gradually around, I can make skin flaps (where skin is separated from underlying breast tissue) up to the clavicle, medially to the sternum, down to the inframammary fold. This is the anatomic extent of the breast tissue.

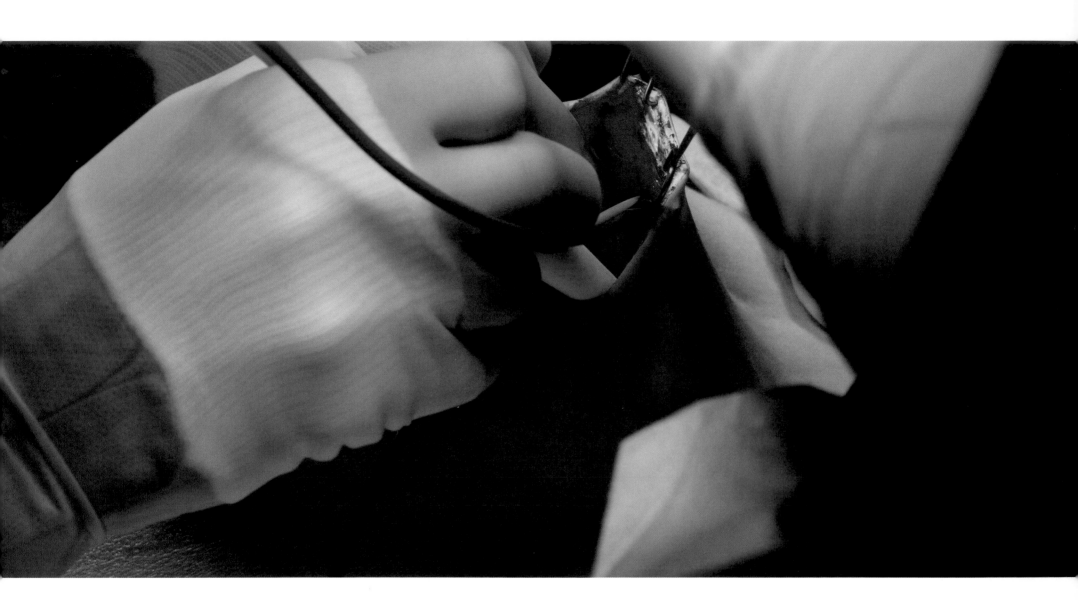

As you can see, there is barely room to work.

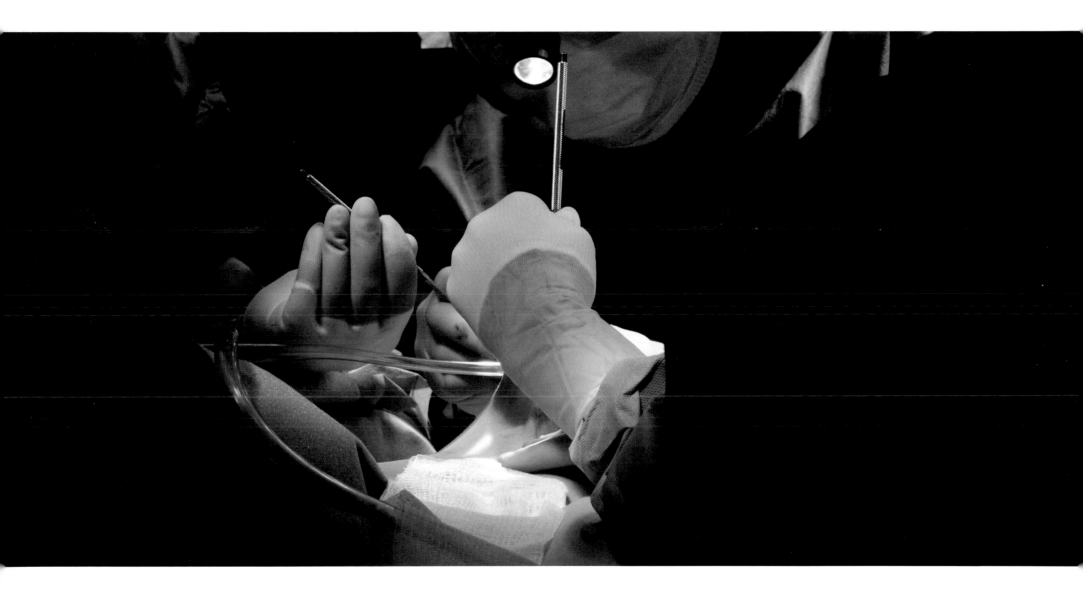

Thus the importance of the head light.

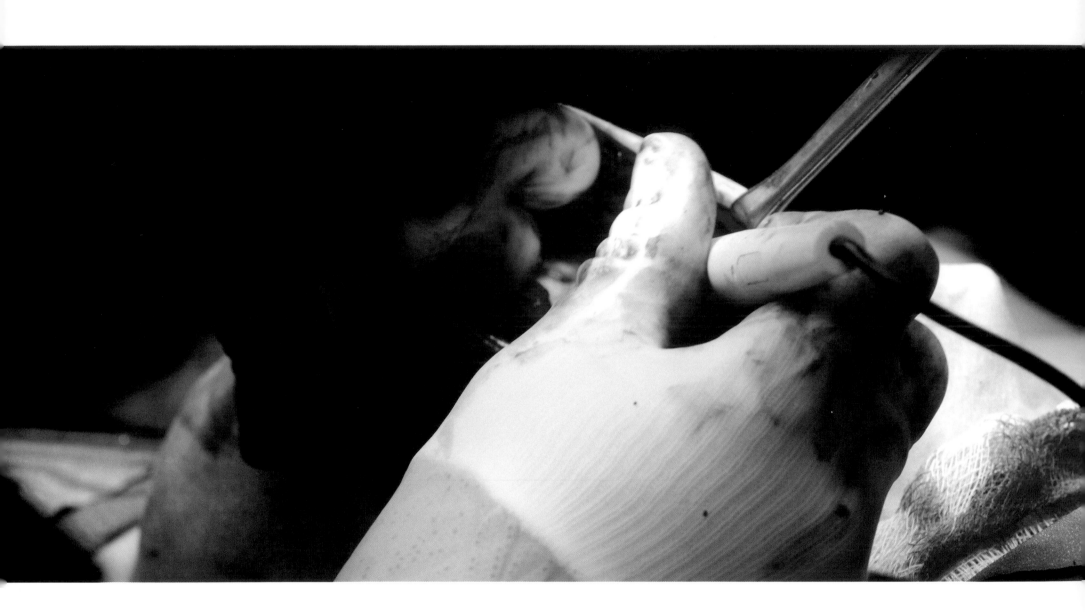

I am continuing my dissection inferiorly. We switch between the skin hooks and a retractor seen in this photo, depending on which provides the best exposure.

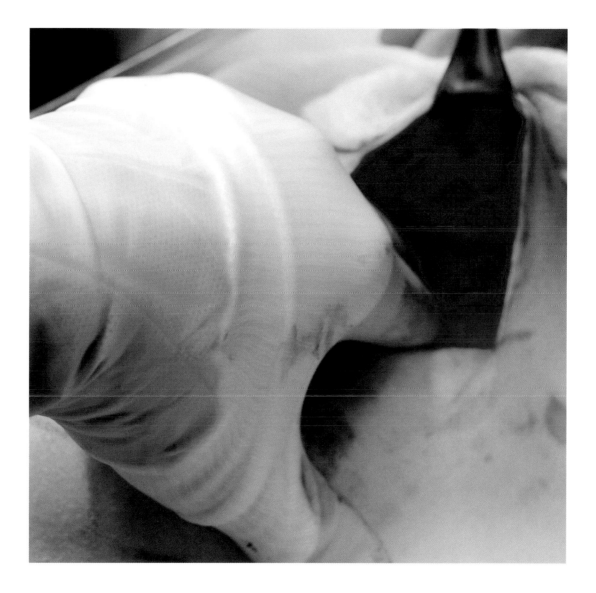

Here I am checking the extent of my flaps.

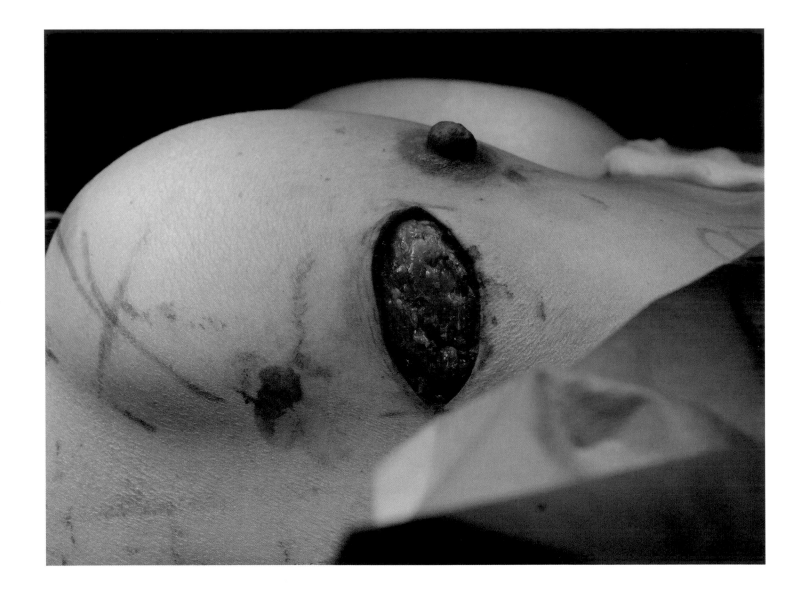

We have completed making the skin flaps and we are taking a rest. This is hard work! Plus, I like to give the skin a rest from all of the pulling.

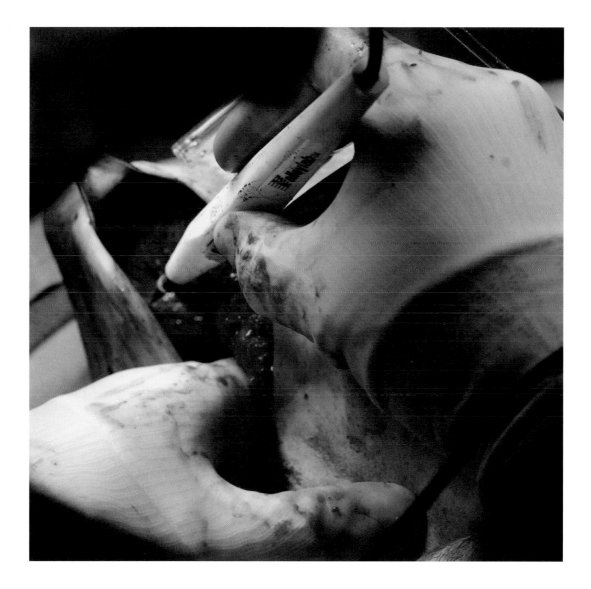

Now, I am in the process of dissecting the breast tissue off the pectoralis muscle fascia.

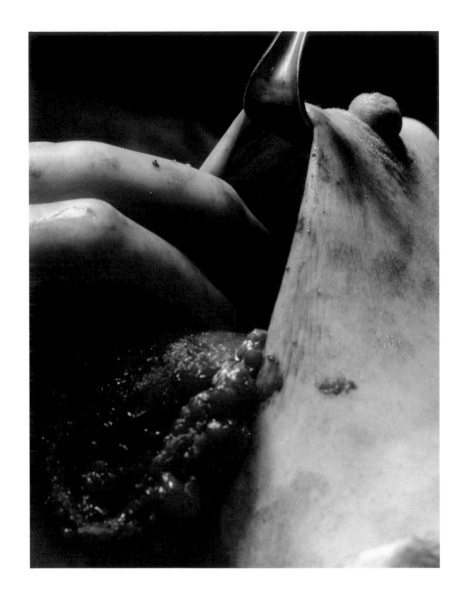

The breast has been dissected partly off the muscle and I have pulled it out of the incision as I continue my dissection.

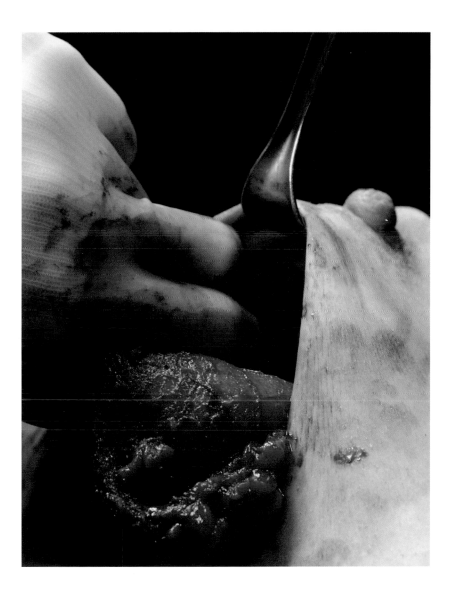

I often pull the breast out then put it back in if I can't get the view I need to continue.

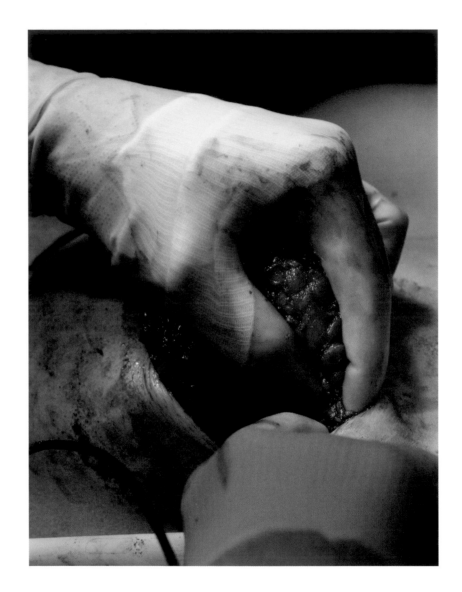

I am carefully dissecting the lateral portion of the breast from the axillary tissue and lateral border of the pectoralis muscle.

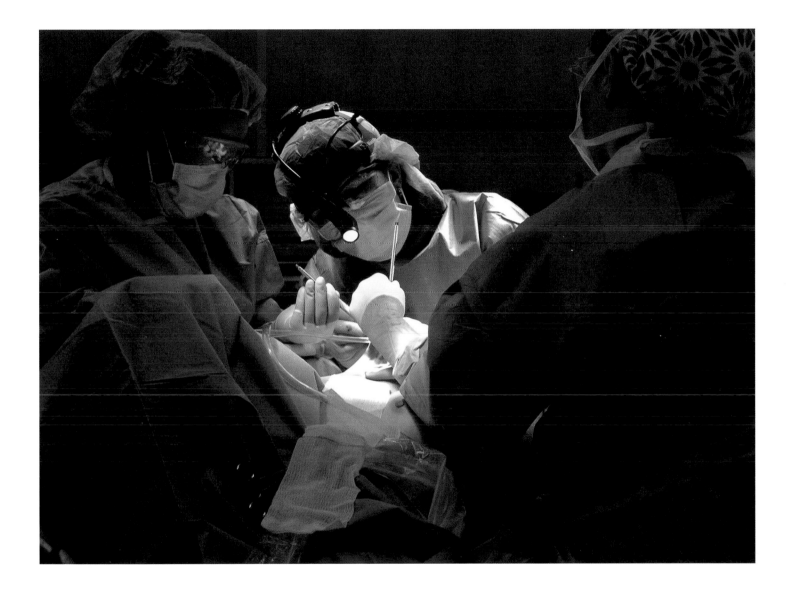

Sometimes a contorted position is required to see the last parts of the dissection.

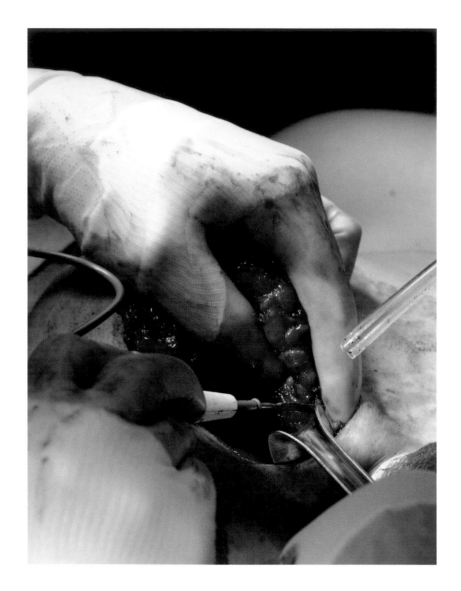

Here I am detaching more of the breast from the skin in the upper outer quadrant.

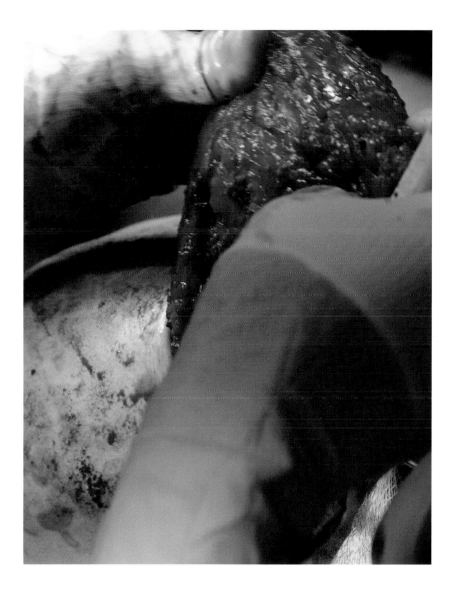

Now the dissection is almost complete. I am pulling the breast out of its skin envelope.

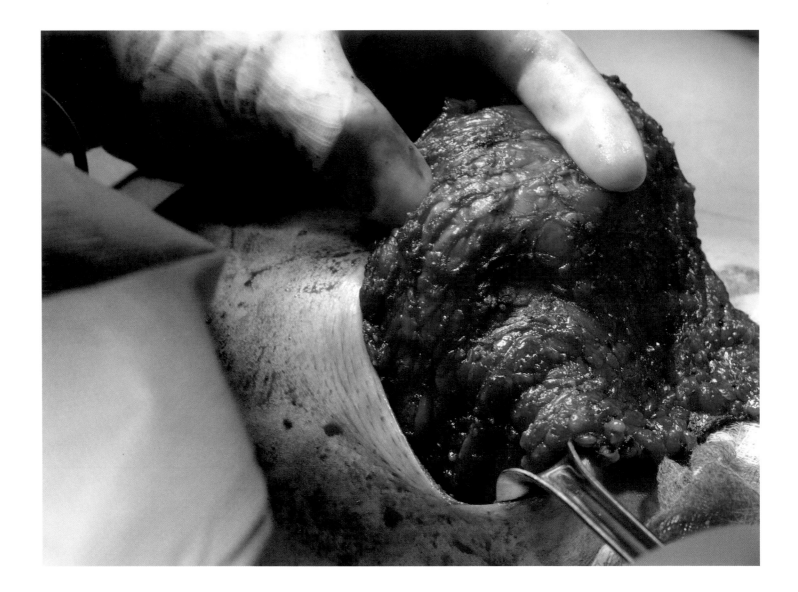

We have laid the breast out on the skin prior to the last part of the dissection so we can orient it for the pathologists.

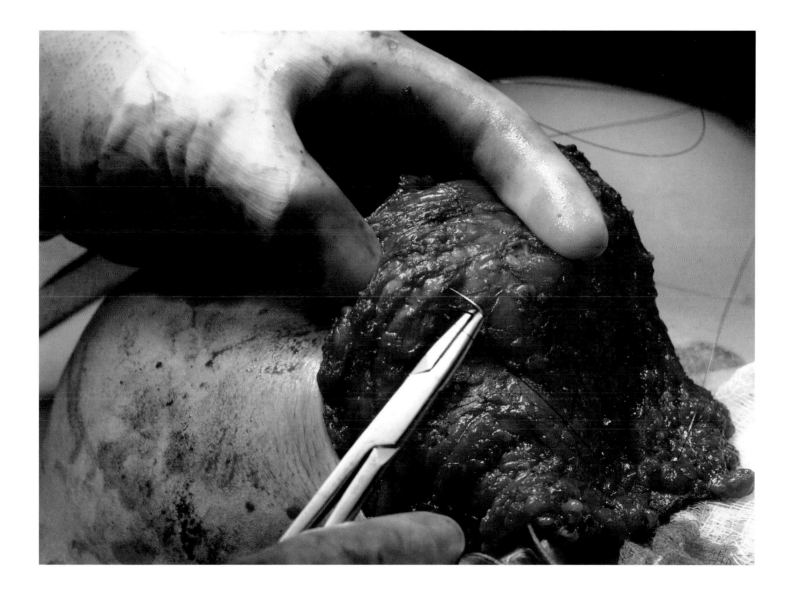

I use the same orientation sutures every time--a blue suture marks the nipple areolar complex, a black suture cut short marks the superior aspect, a black suture cut long marks the lateral aspect.

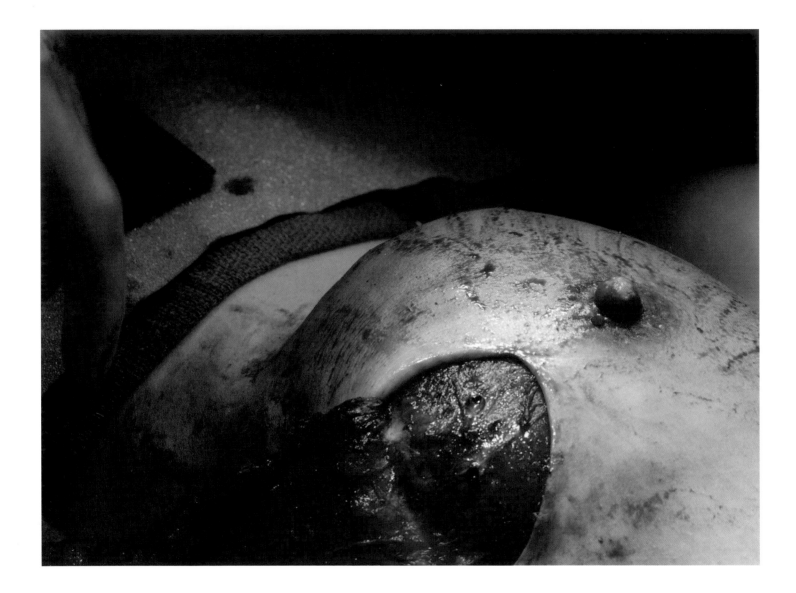

You can see the breast is now only attached at the edge of the muscle.

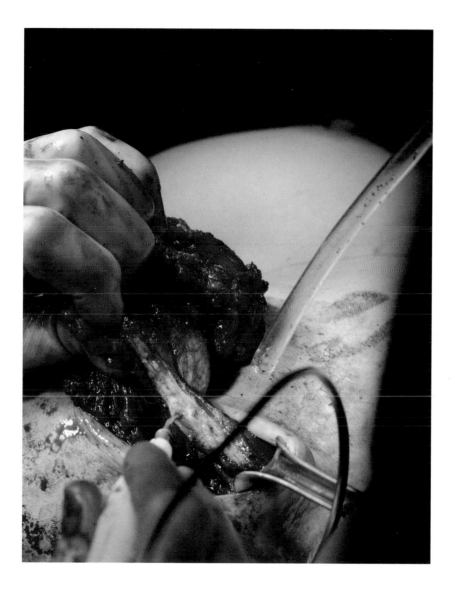

Here I am dissecting the final attachments of the lateral border of the pectoralis muscle.

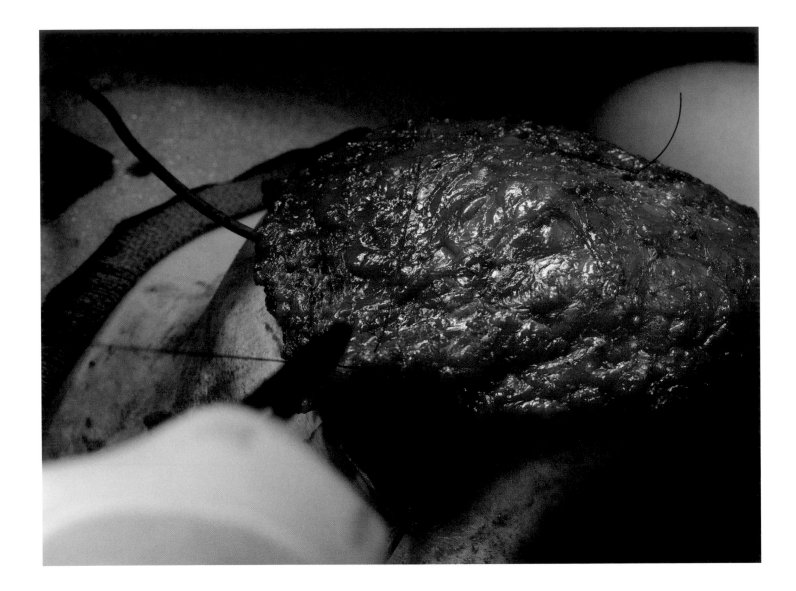

Before we move the breast too far I place that final orientation suture.

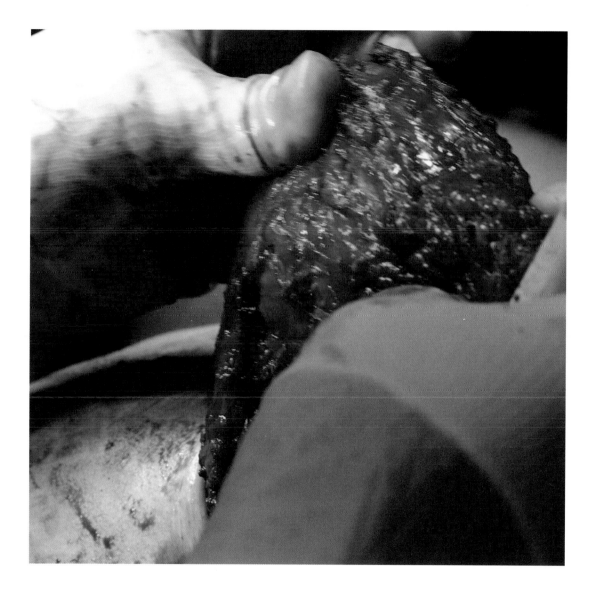

Prior to handing the breast off the field, I palpate it and try to guess how much it weighs (we have a scale in the OR that we use to weigh the breasts. It helps determine what size of expander to use).

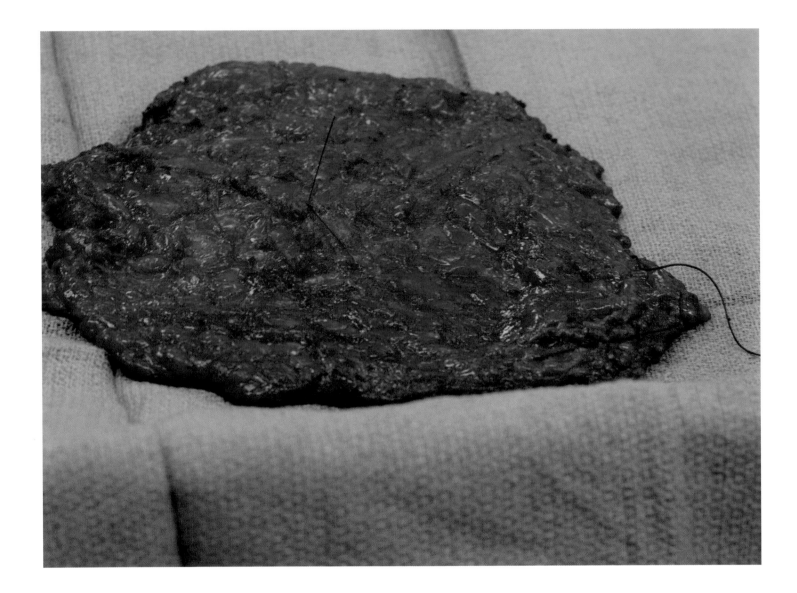

Here is the breast, with the marking sutures.

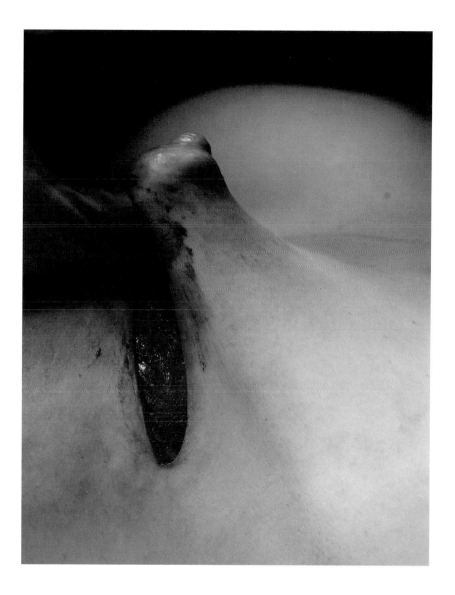

Now I am checking to make sure I have removed as much tissue as possible from under the nipple skin. First I put my fingers under the nipple. Then...

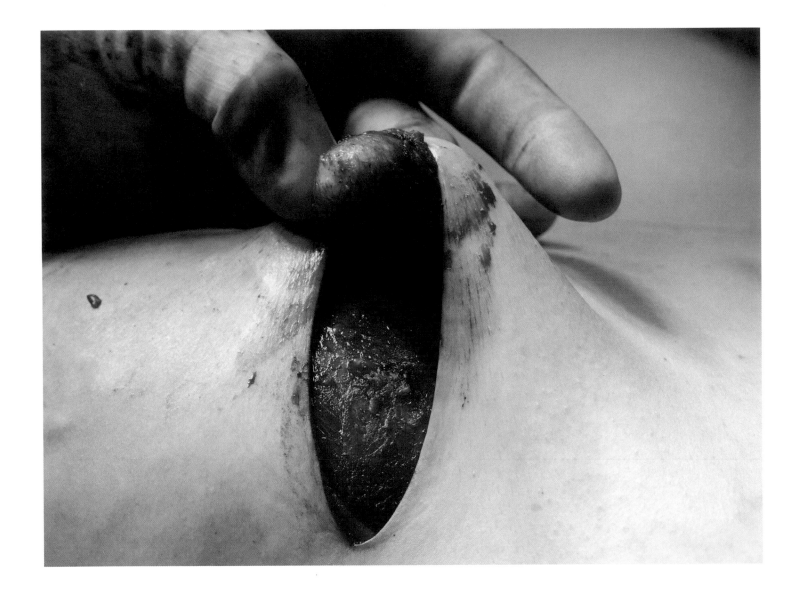

I invert it on my finger to ensure I can only see the underside of the dermis and the cut ends of the ducts.

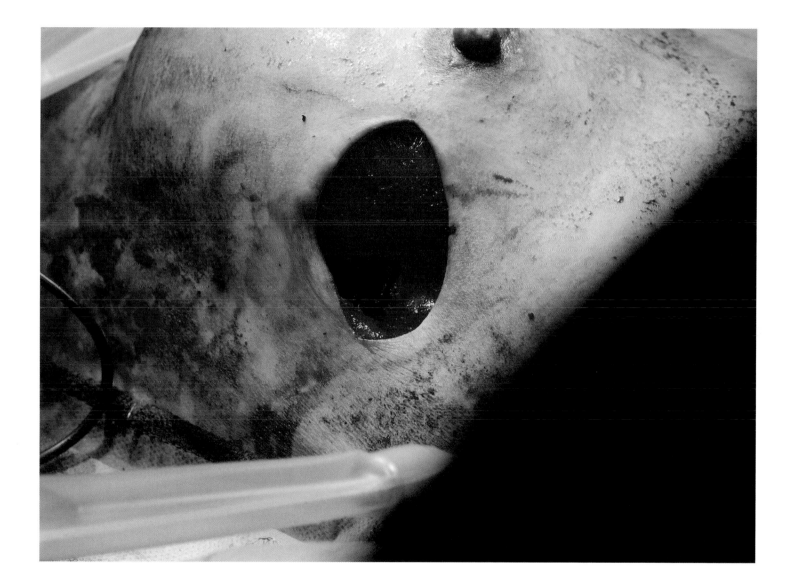

Now it's time to do the sentinel lymph node biopsy. The Geiger counter probe has been covered with a sterile sleeve. I am again looking for the "hot spot," a place where there is enough of the radiolabeled dye collected so that I get activity (both a tone and a number on the screen) on the Geiger counter (R2D2).

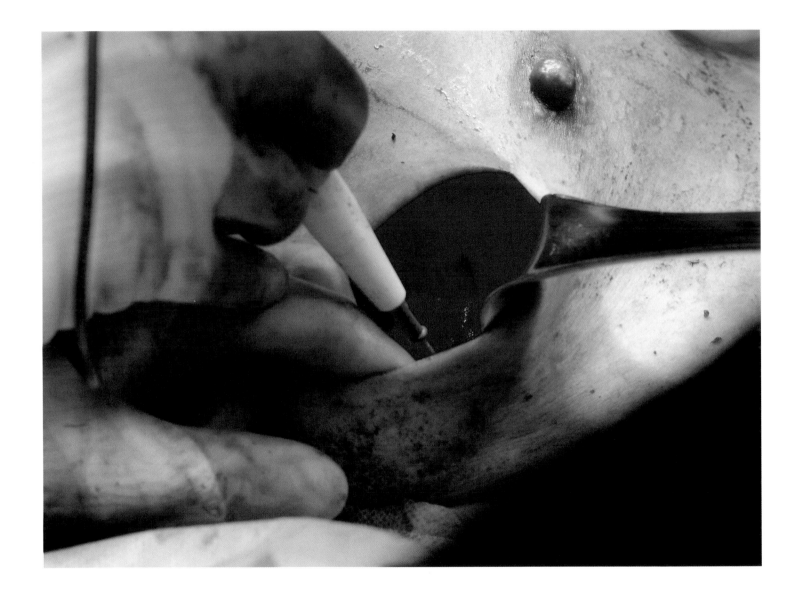

Once I have identified the area with R2D2, I feel for a lymph node and then start to dissect the node away from the surrounding tissue.

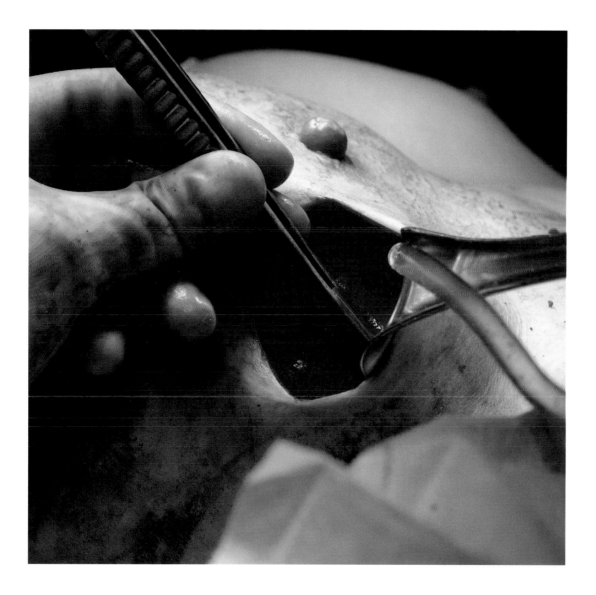

Now I have picked up the node with my forceps to finish the dissection.

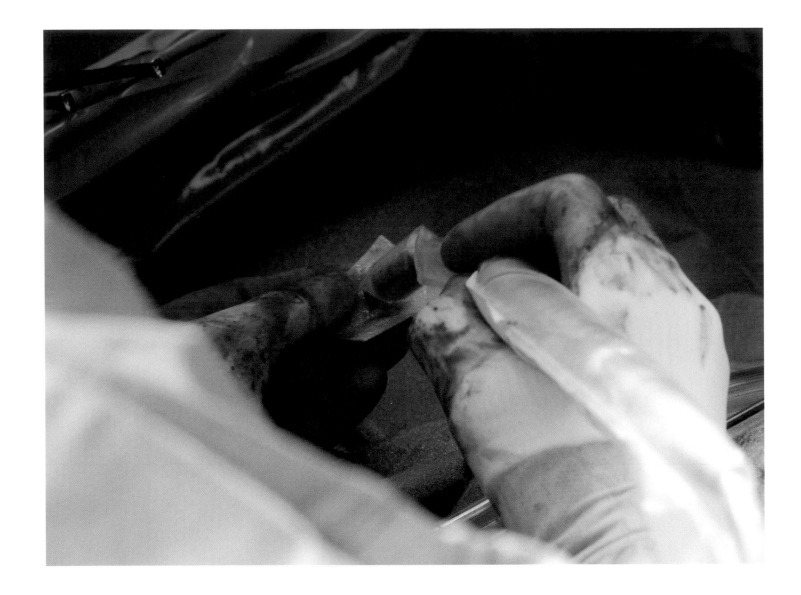

Once the node is out I obtain a "count" with the Geiger counter.

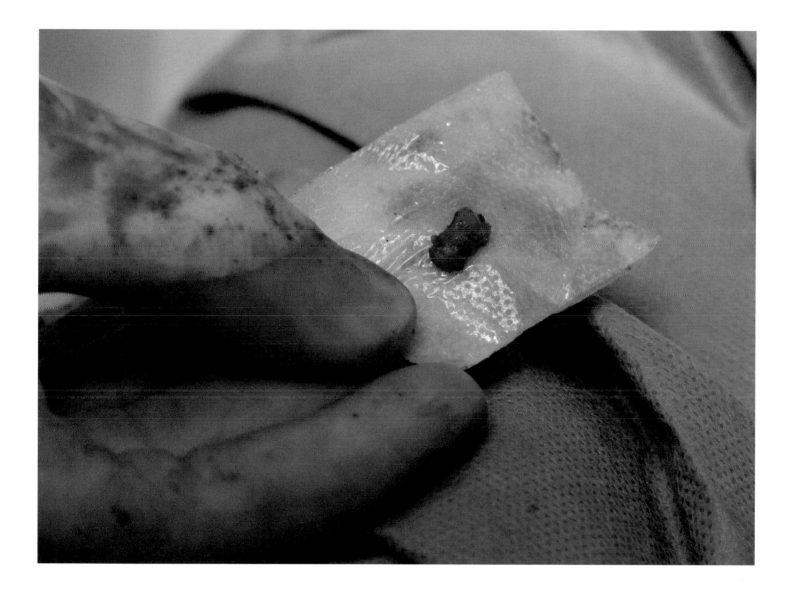

The node is then sent to pathology for analysis.

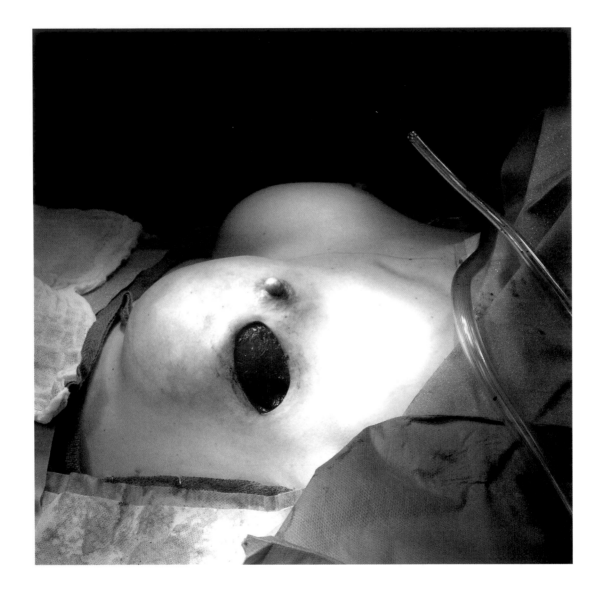

Now that the breast has been removed, we are preparing to remove Shauna's old implant.

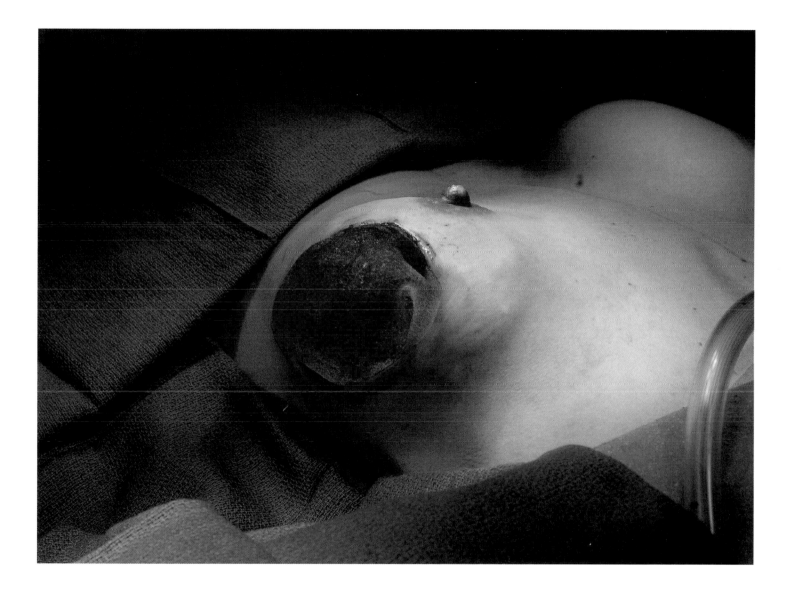

It's halfway out.

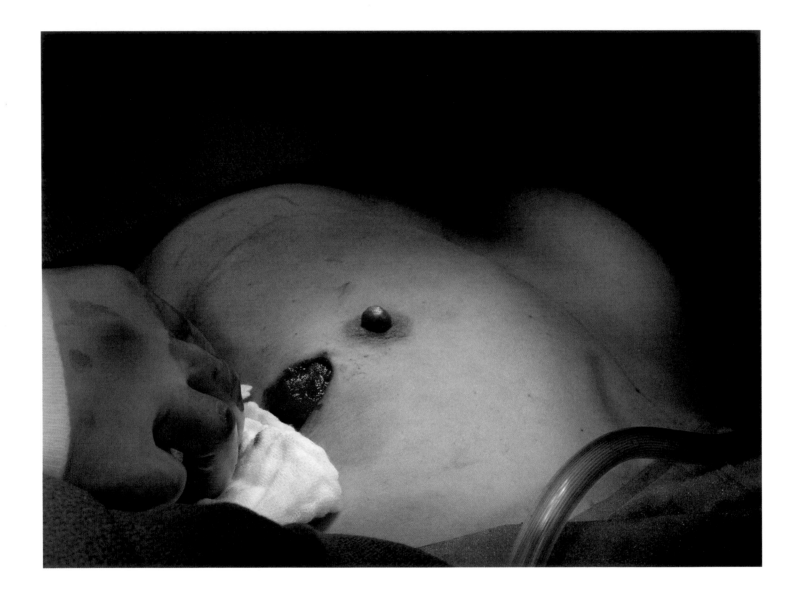

Here is her breast skin after the old implant is out.

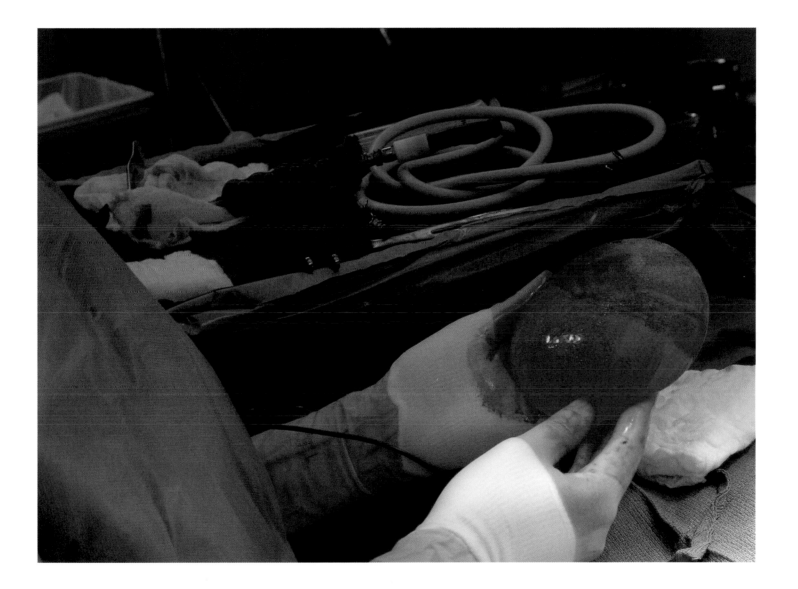

The implant we removed appears intact.

Now Shauna is ready for the reconstructive portion of the surgery with Dr. Agarwal.

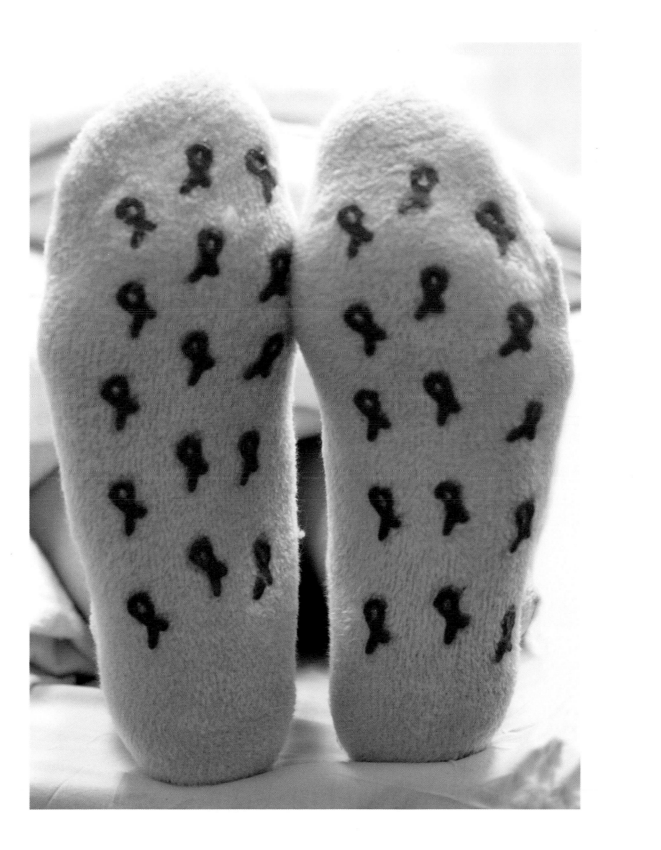

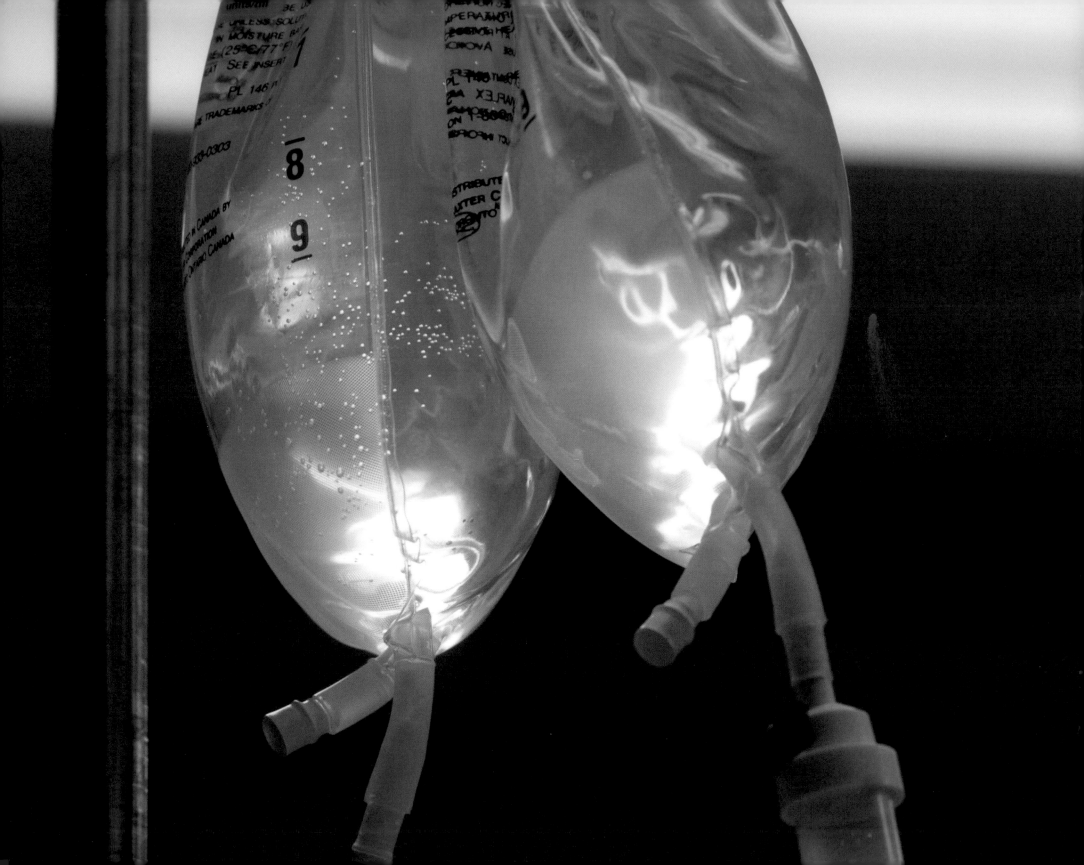

Part 2: Tissue Expander Insertion

The breast reconstruction section shows the surgical sequence of rebuilding a breast after a mastectomy has been performed.

Women with breast cancer fear not only what life will be like after treatment but also what life will be like without breasts. Eight percent of women in the U.S. will be diagnosed with breast cancer in their lifetime. Mastectomy is used to treat 1/3 of the nearly 200,000 women diagnosed with breast cancer annually in the U.S. Recent data suggest that only about 20% of American women undergo breast reconstruction after mastectomy. This low percentage persists despite enactment of the Women's Health and Cancer Rights Act (WHCRA) in 1999, which federally mandates insurance coverage of breast reconstruction.

The primary reason for such an underutilization of post-mastectomy breast reconstruction is lack of education. Patients and their physicians lack knowledge of what options exist for some after a mastectomy. The total care of a patient with breast cancer involves proper diagnosis, medical and oncologic treatment, surgical removal of the cancer, and reconstruction. Breast reconstruction after cancer is no longer a privilege but is an integral component of the comprehensive care of a patient with breast cancer.

The woman shown in these pages was able to undergo a total skin sparing mastectomy. Based on her cancer size and location, all of her skin and her nipple were able to be saved. This is not the case for all women. Her reconstruction involved the use of a tissue expander and was completed with the placement of a breast implant.

There are many techniques for breast reconstruction which include the use of tissue expanders, breast implants or the patient's own tissue. This book highlights one of the most common techniques, which involves a staged approach using both tissue expanders and breast implants.

During the first stage of the reconstruction, the patient has a tissue expander placed in a pocket that is created under the pectoralis major muscle. The expander is a device that can be inflated over time to stretch the skin and pocket to a size suitable for accepting the final implant. We use human cadaver skin to help create the lower half of the pocket. This allows the expander to be completely covered by a layer of tissue in addition to the patient's skin. At the initial stage, blue fluid is used to inflate the expander to begin the expansion process. Only small amounts of fluid are injected into the expander to begin the expansion process, as we don't want additional pressure on the skin from the inside. Additional small amounts of fluid are injected into the expander at each subsequent expansion to allow a gradual stretching of the pocket and skin.

Jay Agarwal, MD

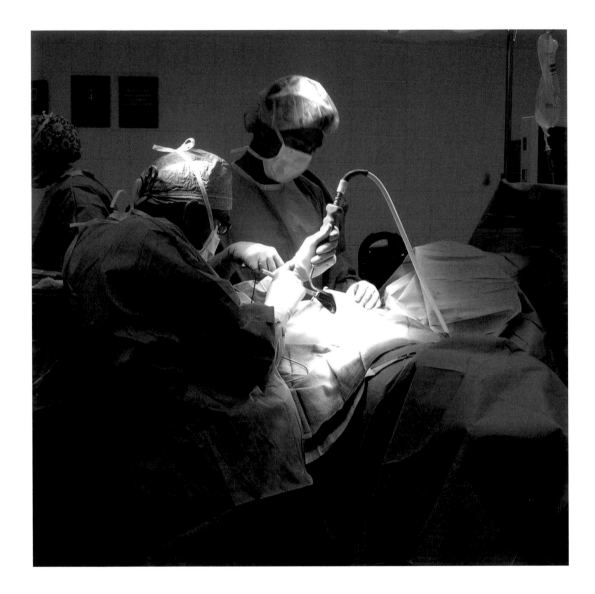

Once the mastectomy has been completed, Dr. Agarwal enters the field and creates a pocket under the chest muscle (pectoralis major). This pocket will be the site of the tissue expander and future implant.

I love Dr. Agarwal's stance in this picture. I can tell he is leaning on me to get the best angle possible. The closeness is really symbolic of the closeness and trust I have for my doctor. It is really important to choose a reconstruction doctor that you can trust by the facts but more important is your own gut instinct. You need to feel they listen to your desires and give you honest feedback about your future. You need to have an "I feel really good about my doctor" experience.

87

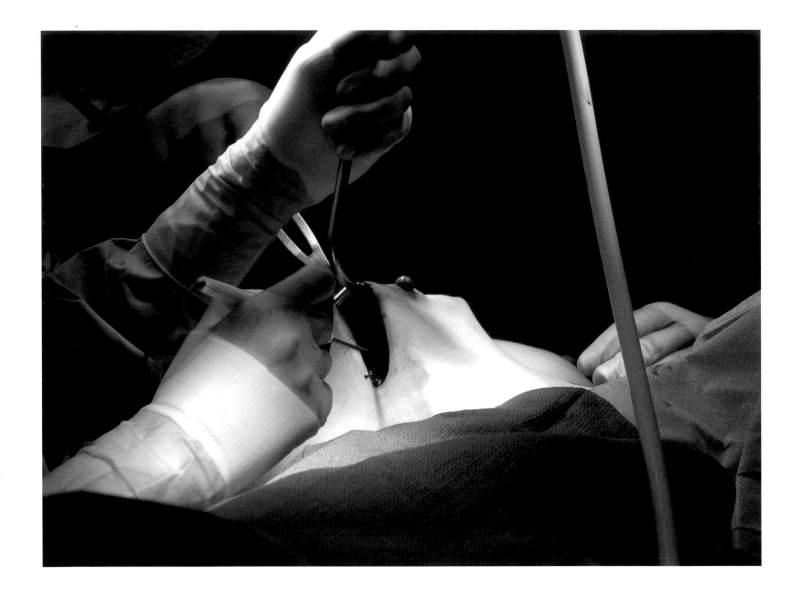

We use a hand held cautery device to help create the pocket. This device also helps control bleeding.

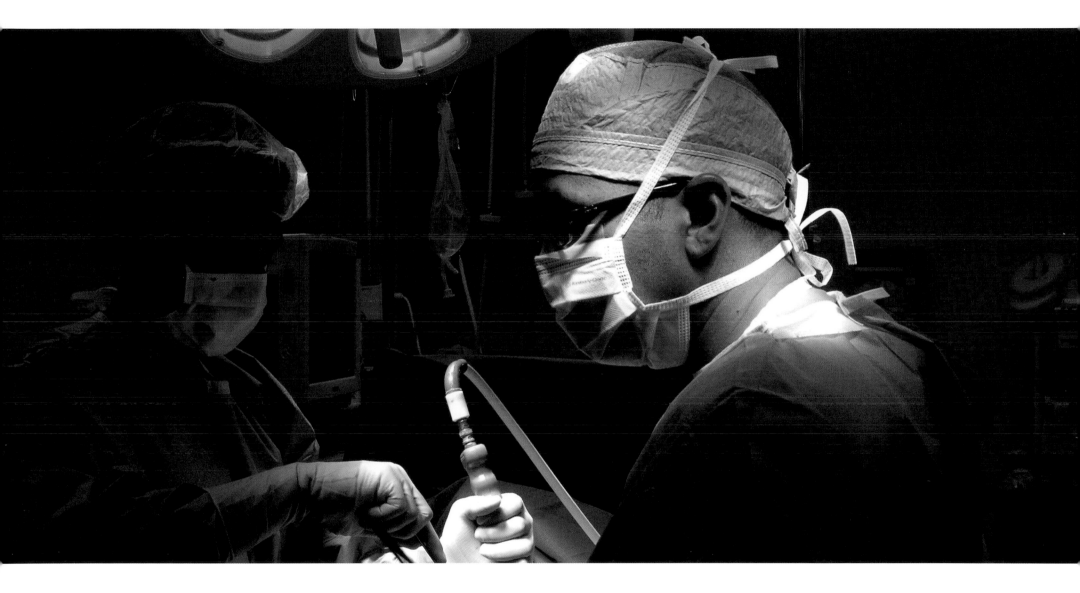

My assistant (left in photo) helps me see by holding the incision open.

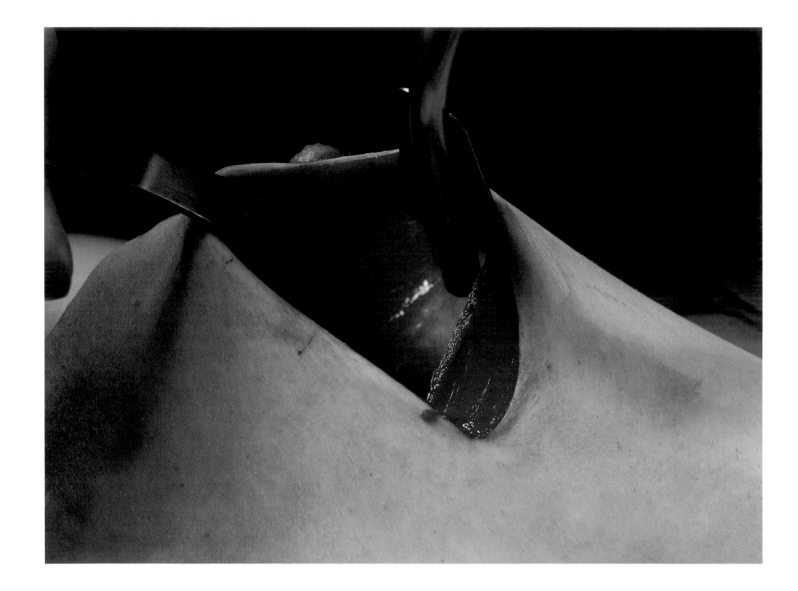

The instrument on the right of the photo (retractor) lifts up the pectroalis major muscle, showing the pocket we have created.

The cavern of my empty breast is like the darkness of my spirit at hearing the diagnosis of cancer. You are so unsure of the true diagnosis until the actual surgery and dissection. I chose immediate reconstruction because I wanted the emotional transition of losing a breast to be easier.

It was easier.

I liked looking down at my little expander after waking up from the surgery.

91

92

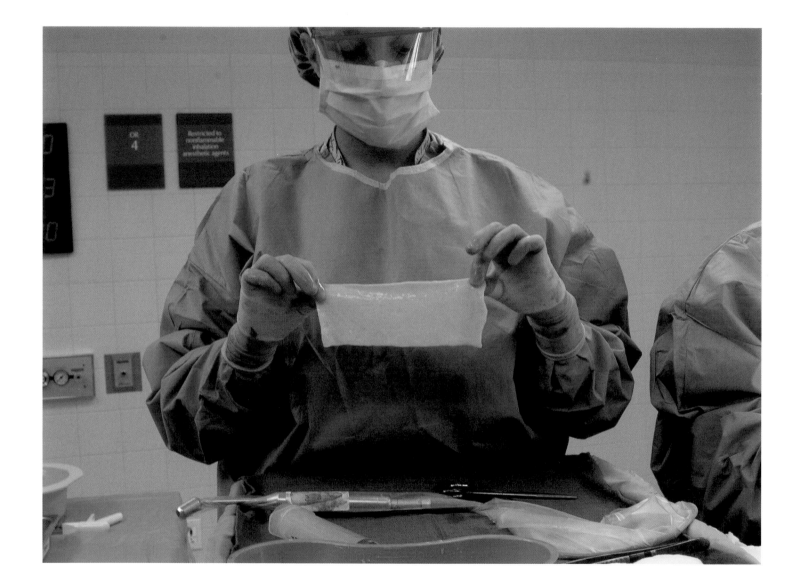

We use human cadaver skin to create a sling for the expander. This provides an extra layer (in addition to the breast skin) on the side and bottom of the cavity where muscle isn't available.

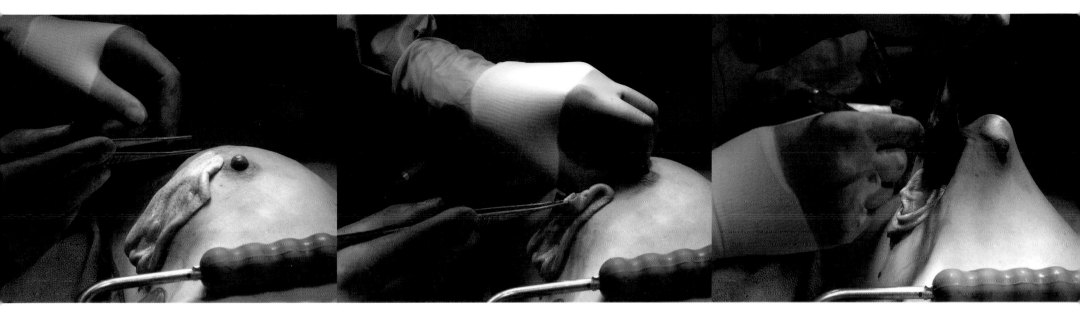

We place the cadaver skin into the breast cavity and stitch it to the muscle and along the lower edge of the cavity to create the lower part of the pocket.

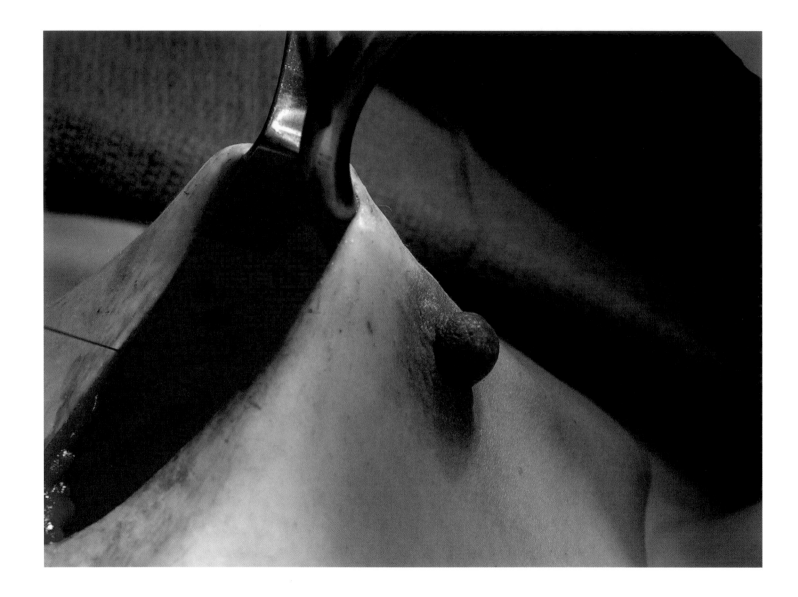

We have placed the first stitch to secure the cadaver skin.

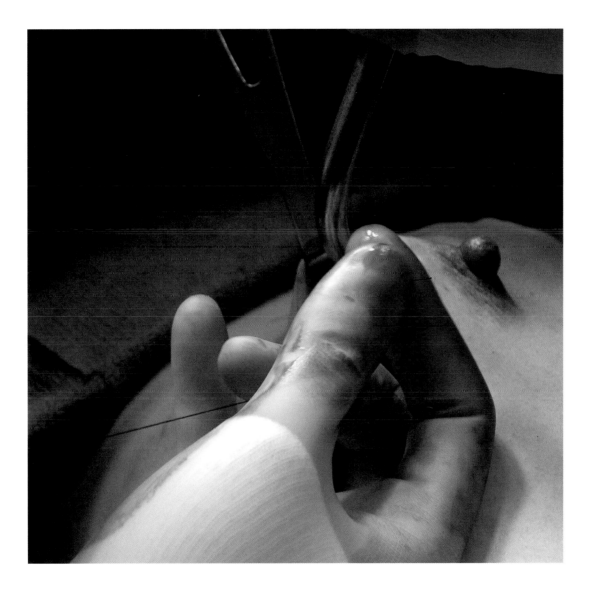

Now I tie the first knot.

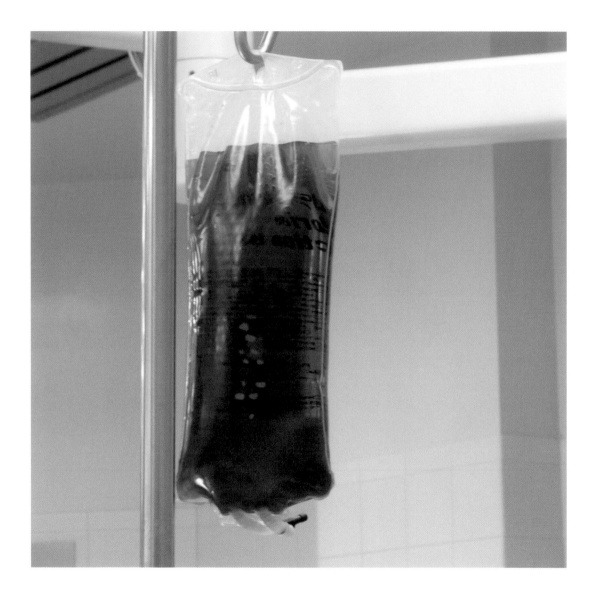

We use blue colored water to fill the tissue expander. The blue color helps us make sure we are in the right place when we add fluid later in the clinic.

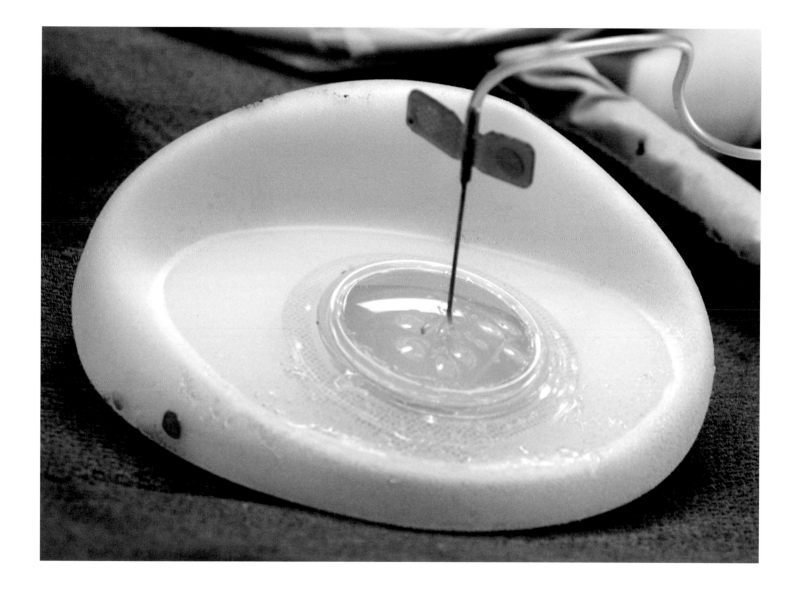

First, we prepare the tissue expander by deflating it of all air.

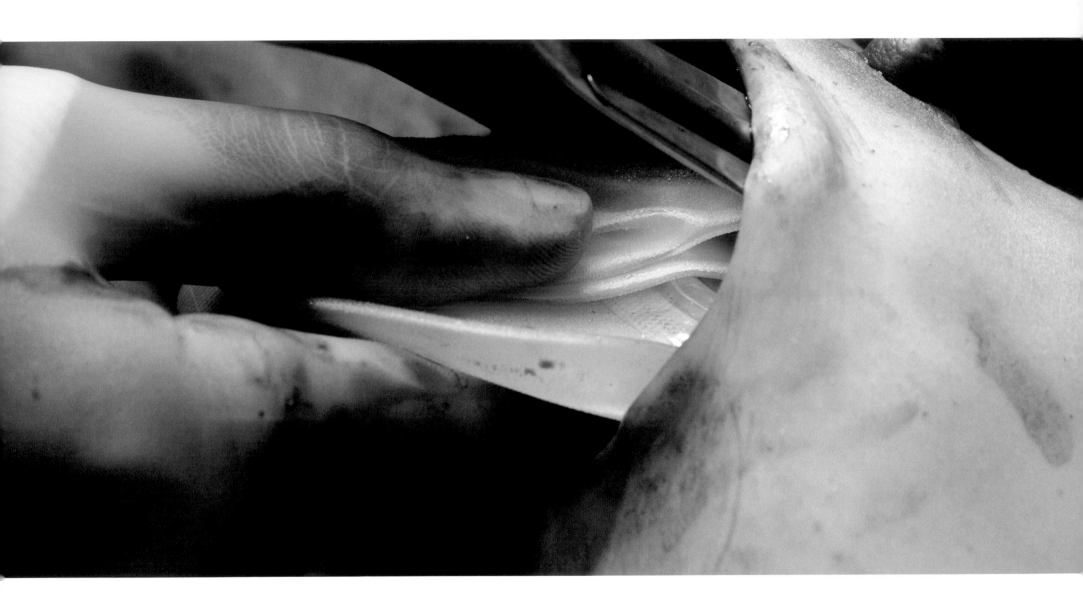

In order to get the tissue expander in through our small incision, we have to fold it so we can place it in the pocket we have made under the pectoralis (chest) muscle.

This reminds me of inserting a soft shoe insole. It's a tricky procedure making sure you get it in right so it doesn't bunch under the ball of your foot. I can only imagine what a challenge a breast would be.

100

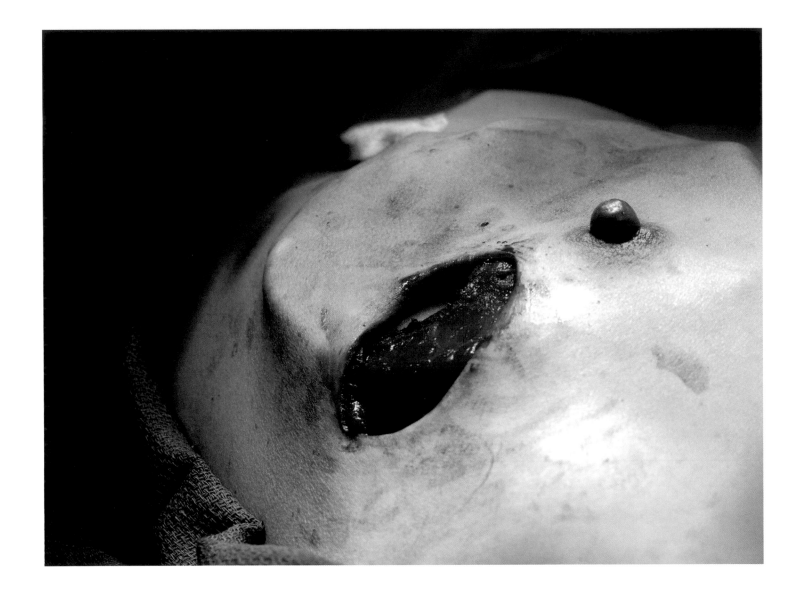

We can see the tissue expander in the pocket through an opening between the chest muscle (pectoralis major) and the cadaver skin.

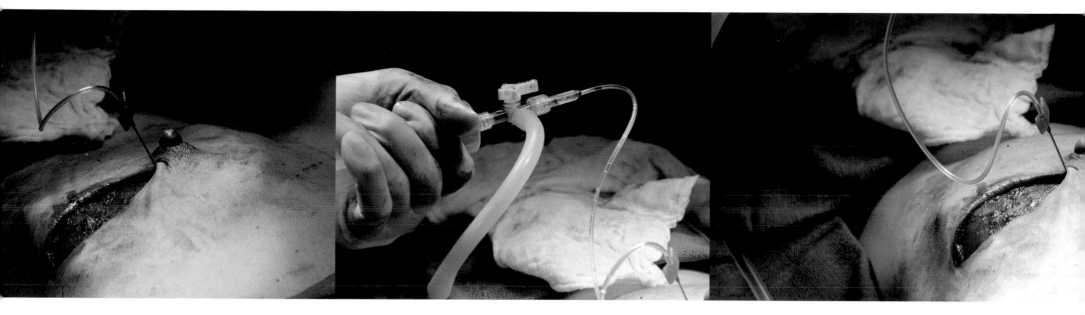

We are now injecting the blue fluid into the tissue expander.

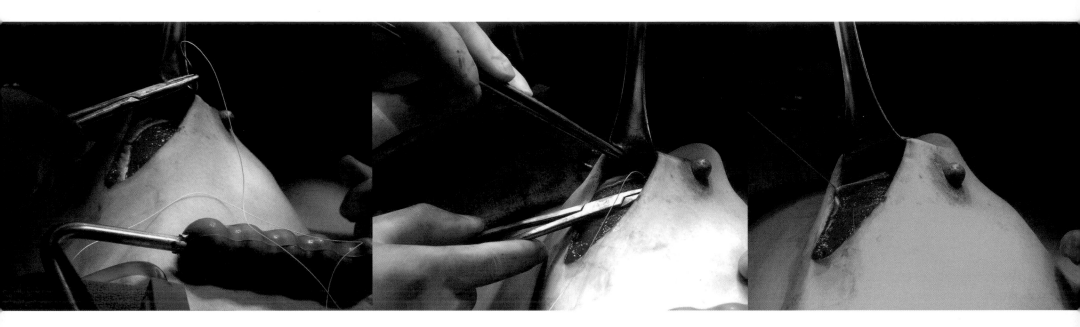

Once I have partially filled the expander, I stitch the edge of the pectoralis muscle to the cadaver skin to completely enclose the expander.

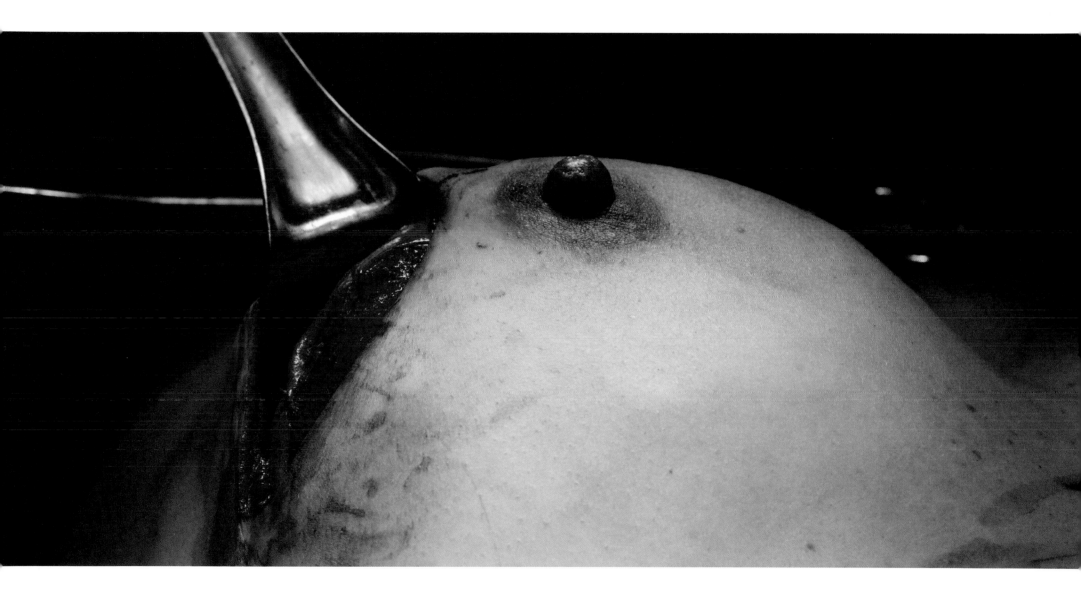

We put enough fluid in to start to give the shape of a new breast. I don't fill it all the way since that could put pressure on the skin from the inside.

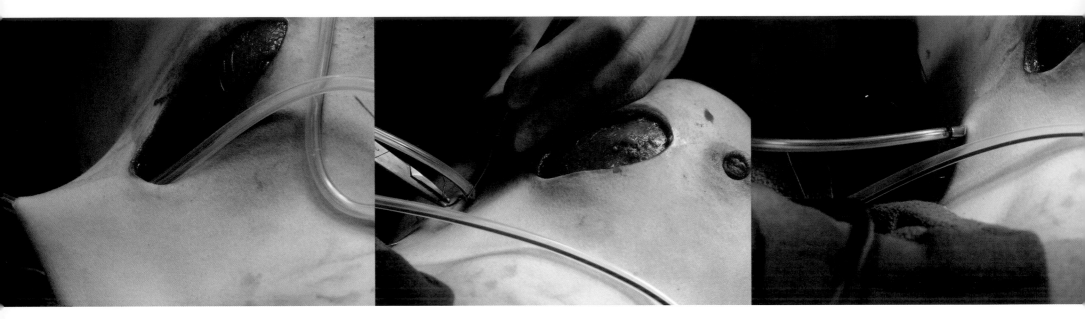

Here I am inserting a drainage tube. It is brought out through a separate incision in the low armpit. I sew it in because it will need to stay in for a couple of weeks.

It's so fascinating to see my muscle wall so clean, red and beautiful, my breast no longer housing a potential killer. It's amazing how stretchy the skin is here as well. It reminds me of the resiliency we have as women to overcome challenges.

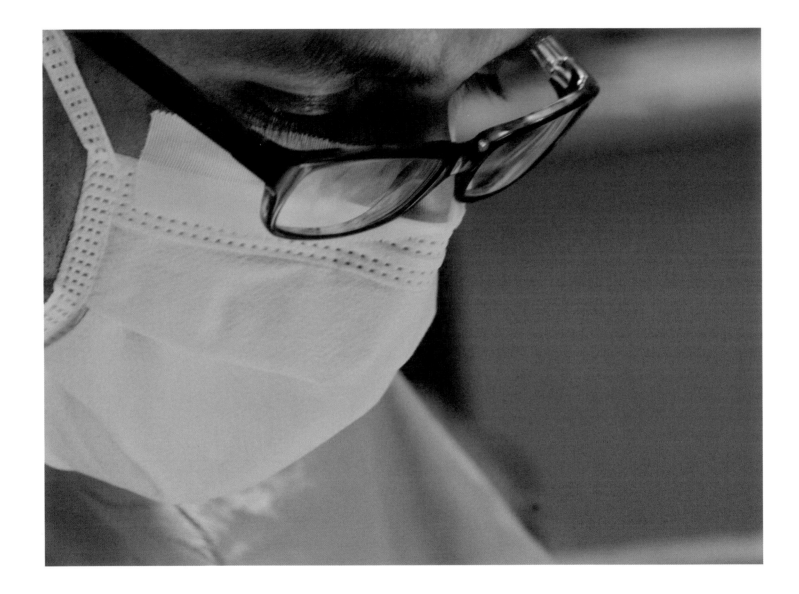

Here I am checking the size and position of the expander. The tape on the top of my mask helps to keep my glasses from fogging.

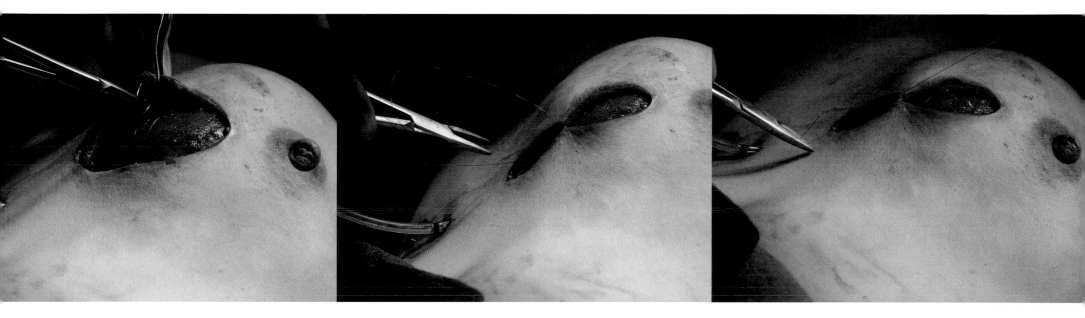

I am starting to close the skin. I first put several stitches in the deep layer of the skin.

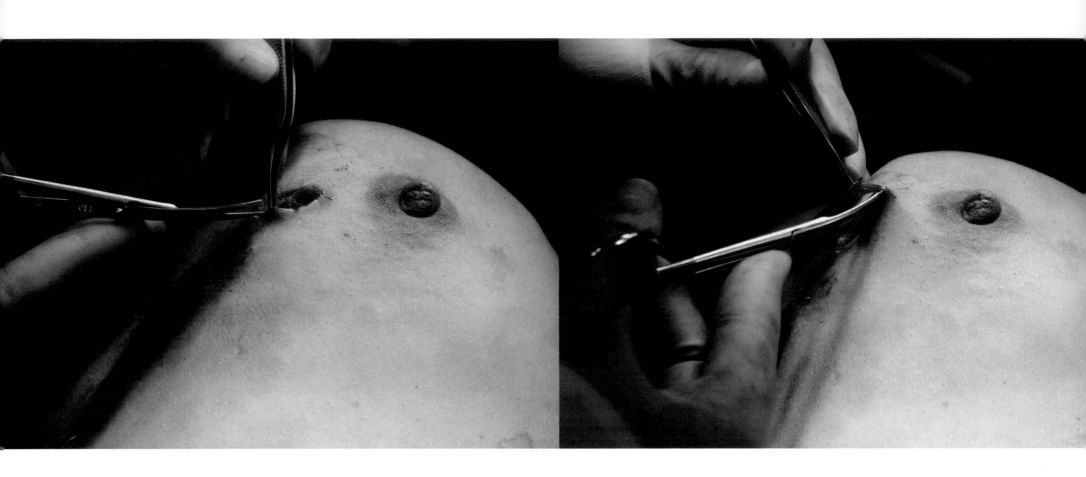

I trim the skin edges to make them fit together nicely.

I am amazed by the fine tuning skills my surgeon has here. This is the most challenging patchwork quilt, putting me back together again. I felt like this procedure was the little extra gift suggested by my surgeon, which will give me the best outcome.

Reconstruction was never a question for me. When I first met Dr. Agarwal, my reconstruction doctor, I told him I wanted reconstruction to be the gift after the heartache of cancer. I suggest asking your surgeon all the possibilities, because there are so many now.

Part 3: Permanent Implant Insertion

The permanent implant insertion section of *Meet Virginia* finishes showing the surgical sequence of rebuilding a breast after a mastectomy has been performed. Although there are many ways to reconstruct the breast, this section takes the reader through one of the most common techniques and provides a reasonable overview of what can be expected.

111

Permanent Implant Insertion

This section of *Meet Virginia* depicts Shauna Smith as she continues through her reconstructive process. She periodically returns to Dr. Agarwal's office for inflation of the tissue expander. Once she reaches a size that both she and her surgeon are comfortable with, planning for the final reconstruction begins.

It is important to remember that Shauna did not require chemotherapy or radiation. When patients require chemotherapy and/or radiation, the time frame from diagnosis to final reconstruction may be as long as a year. There are many different ways to reconstruct a breast. In some cases we are able to use implants for the final reconstruction; however if there is not enough breast skin or if the skin is fragile, we often have to borrow tissue from another part of the body to rebuild the breast. In Shauna's case, her tissues were healthy enough to allow her to have an implant based reconstruction.

After the completion of her expansion, Shauna discusses with Dr. Agarwal the type of implant to use, saline or silicone. During this surgery, Shauna will have her tissue expander removed from her treated breast and an implant placed in the pocket created under her pectoralis muscle. Also, Shauna will have her old breast implant removed from her untreated breast and a new implant will be placed in that breast to achieve symmetry. Finally, small adjustments to the shape and position of her breasts on her chest wall will be made to achieve the best possible outcome.

A bit about implants:

Although we use the same breast implants for cosmetic augmentation as we do in breast reconstruction after mastectomy, it is very important to understand that the appearance, the feel, and the outcomes are very different. After mastectomy, the healing properties of the chest wall are different than in a person who hasn't undergone prior breast surgery. Therefore, the potential complications and outcomes after breast reconstruction are different than after a cosmetic breast augmentation.

A woman undergoing breast reconstruction with implants will ultimately have to decide whether to have silicone implants or saline implants placed. Both of these implants have the potential for infection and leakage and both can develop capsular contracture, which is a hardening and tightening of the tissue around the implant that may develop and result in a painful, tightened, or irregularly shaped breast.

There has been controversy and investigation into the safety of silicone breast implants. The FDA, physicians and private industry have studied the effects of silicone breast implants in women after augmentation or in reconstruction. Currently, silicone implants are available to women of all ages for breast reconstruction and women aged 22 years and older for breast augmentation. It appears, from these investigations, that the fears of developing autoimmune disease from silicone breast implants may be unfounded. However, it must be understood that the medical community does not know everything there is to know about silicone implants. Long term studies continue and as new information becomes available, it will be conveyed to patients.

114

The safest practice for any woman contemplating breast implants, whether for cosmetic augmentation or for breast reconstruction, is to consult her plastic surgeon and obtain information from the American Society of Plastic Surgeons.

Jay Agarwal, MD

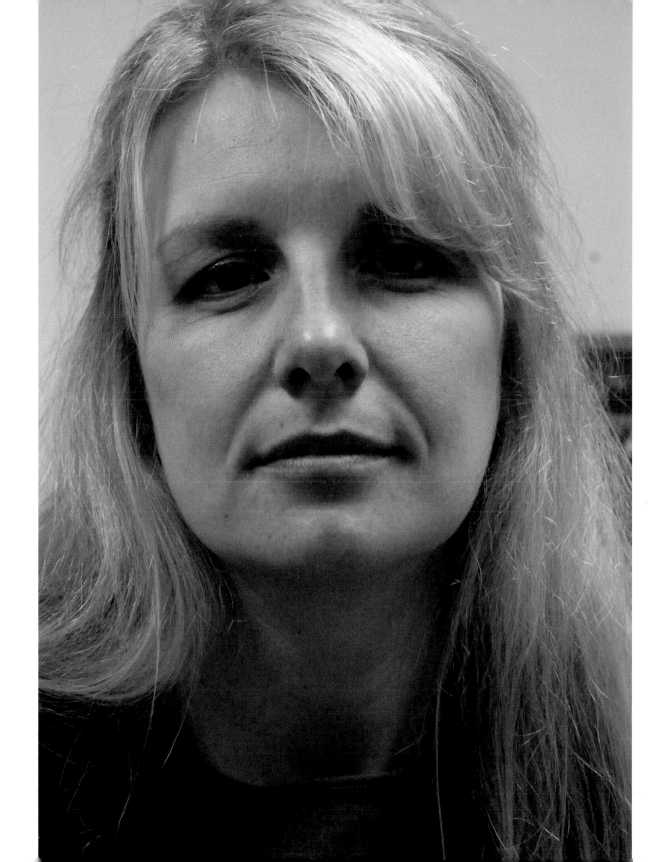

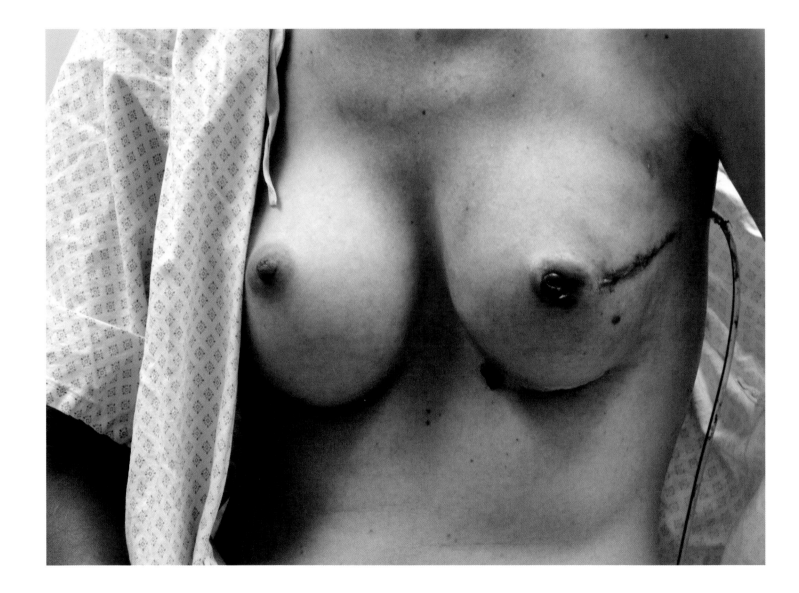

At her first clinic visit, Shauna has some bruising and discoloration of her breast and nipple.

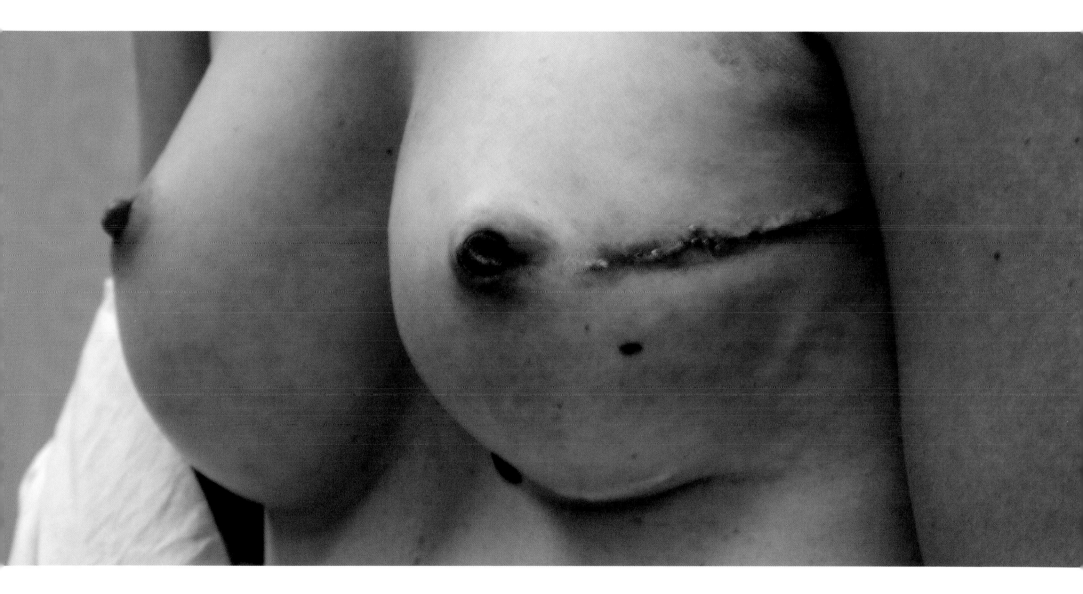

The incision on the side of her breast is healing appropriately.

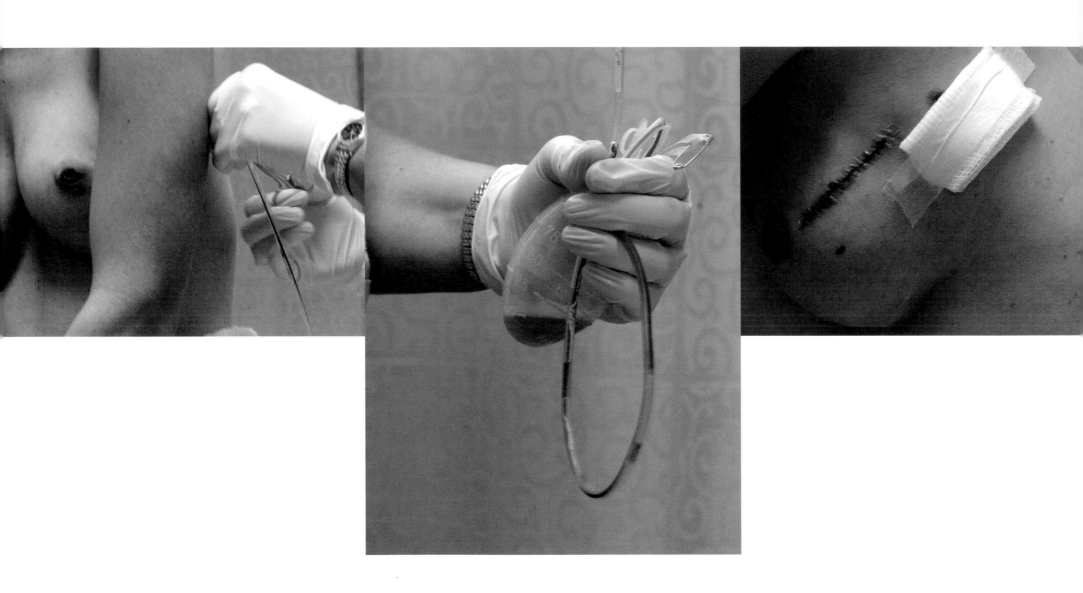

We usually are able to remove the drains 1-2 weeks after surgery. The output is yellowish (plasma) or can be bloody. We apply a gauze pad to the drain hole.

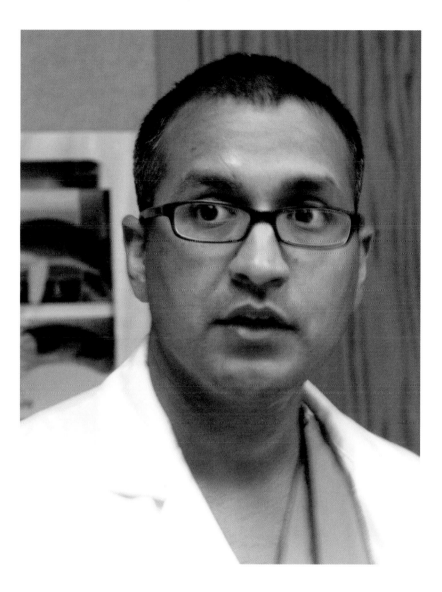

I explain the plan for subsequent expansions to Shauna.

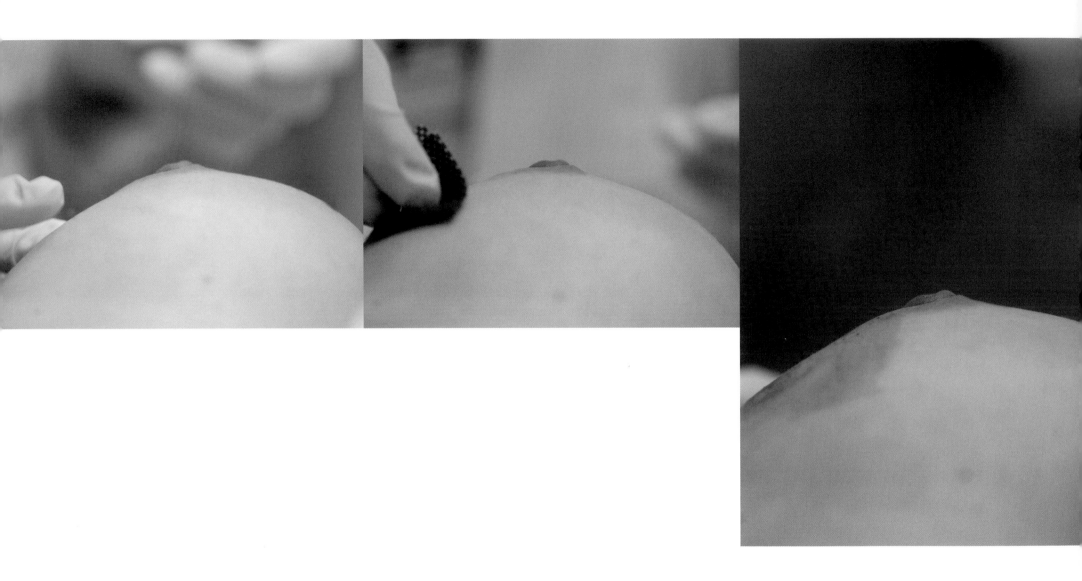

Over a number of weeks, we slowly inflate the expander by adding small amounts of fluid. This is done to stretch the skin and muscle in anticipation of the final reconstruction.

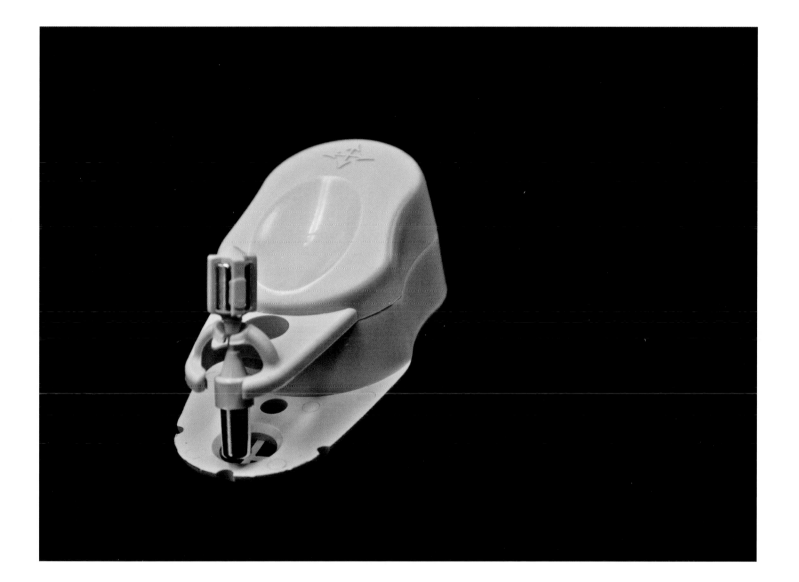

We use a magnet to locate the entry port for filling up Shauna's expander. Although it looks huge here, in real life it is about two inches long.

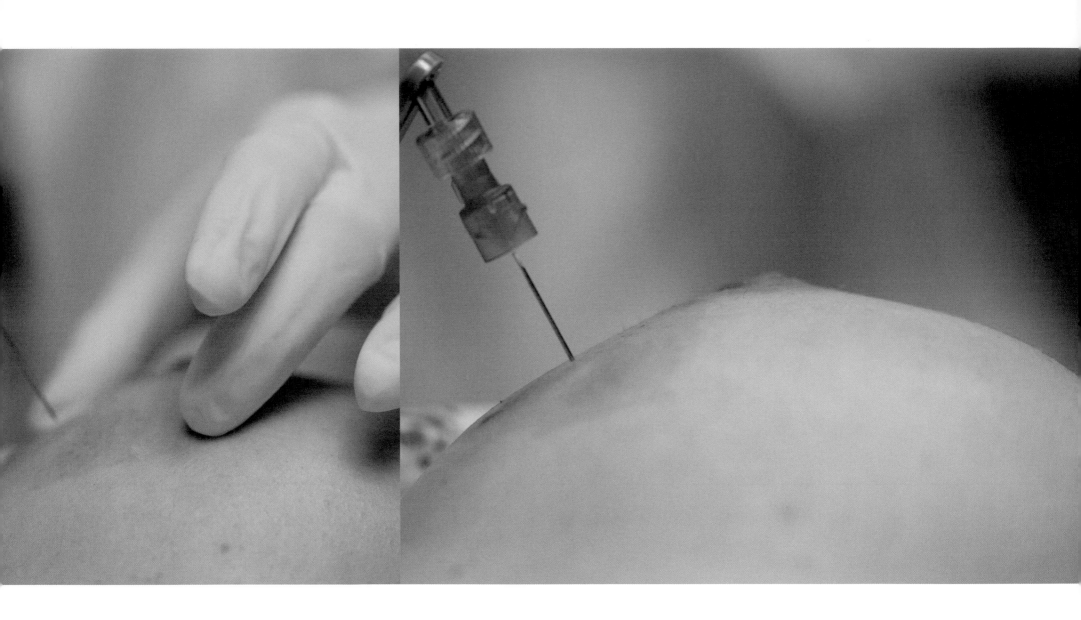

We clean the skin with Betadine and insert a needle into the port to instill saline into the expander.

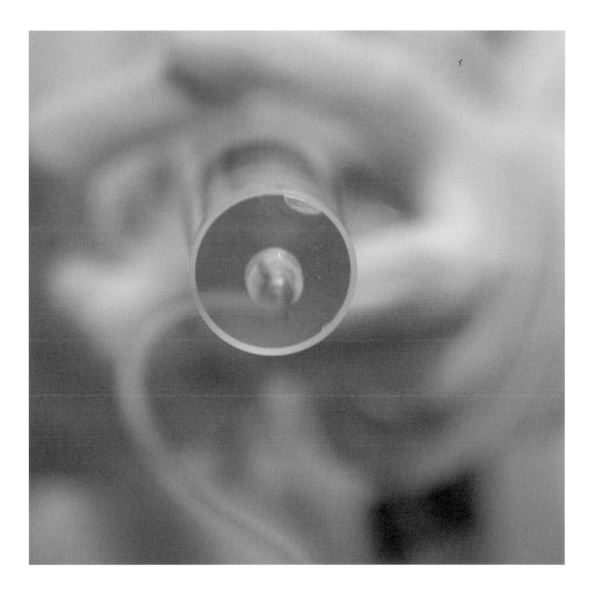

Shauna's perspective as she is expanded.

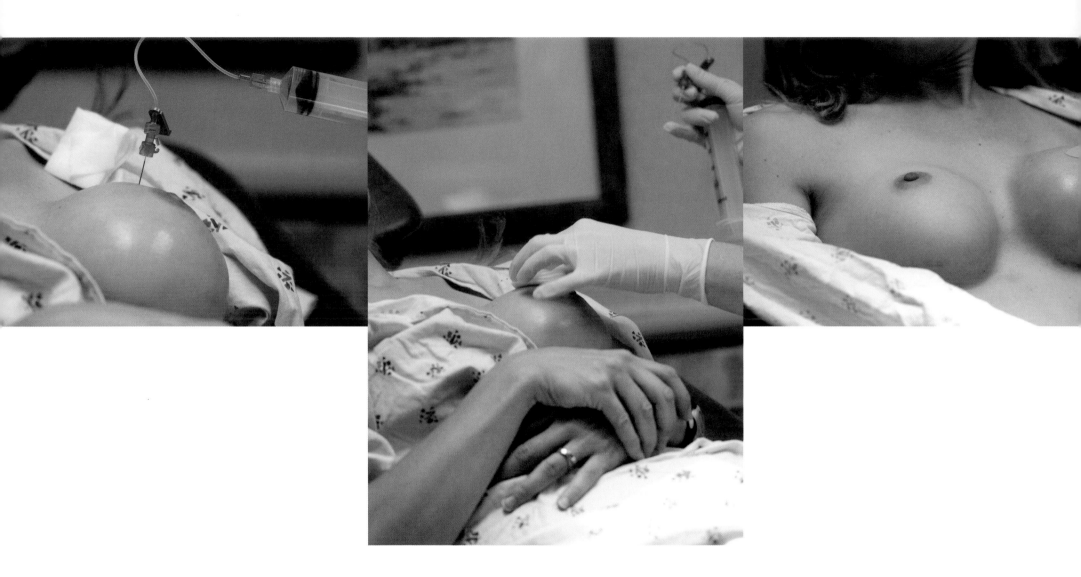

Only about 60-100 cc (2-3 ounces) are instilled into the expander every week or two to gradually stretch the breast skin and chest muscle.

The plan for the next surgery has been discussed with Shauna. We are going to remove the tissue expander from her left breast by going through her mastectomy incision. A permanent silicone implant will then be placed in the pocket (under her pectoralis muscle).

On her right side, Shauna has a pre-existing permanent implant which we will replace with a new implant to match the newly reconstructed left side. Additionally, we will reposition the implants so that her nipples are more centered on her breasts.

125

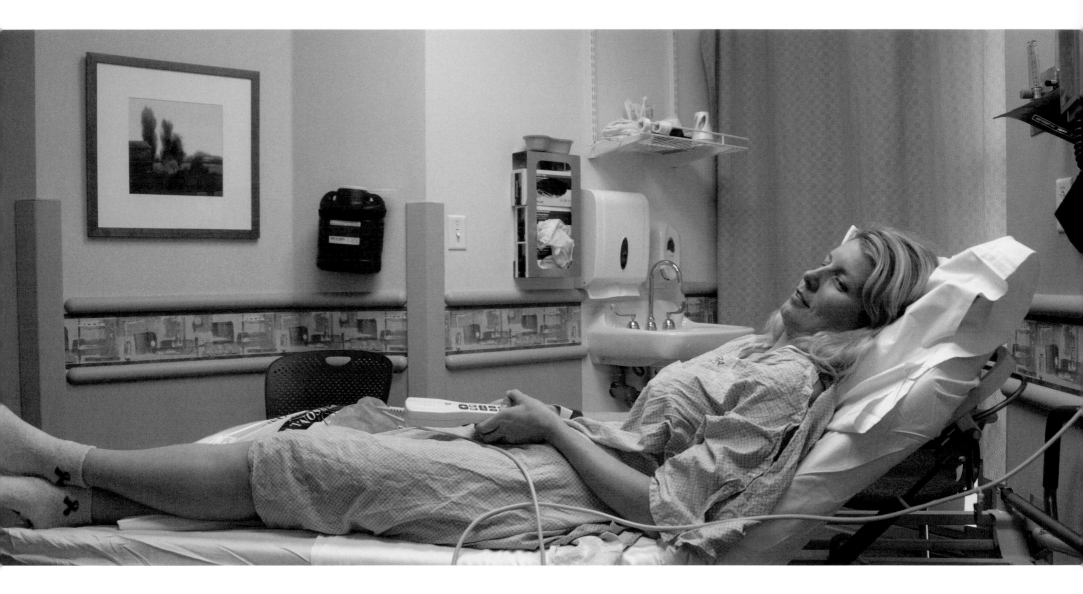

Shauna distracts herself before the final surgery by watching TV.

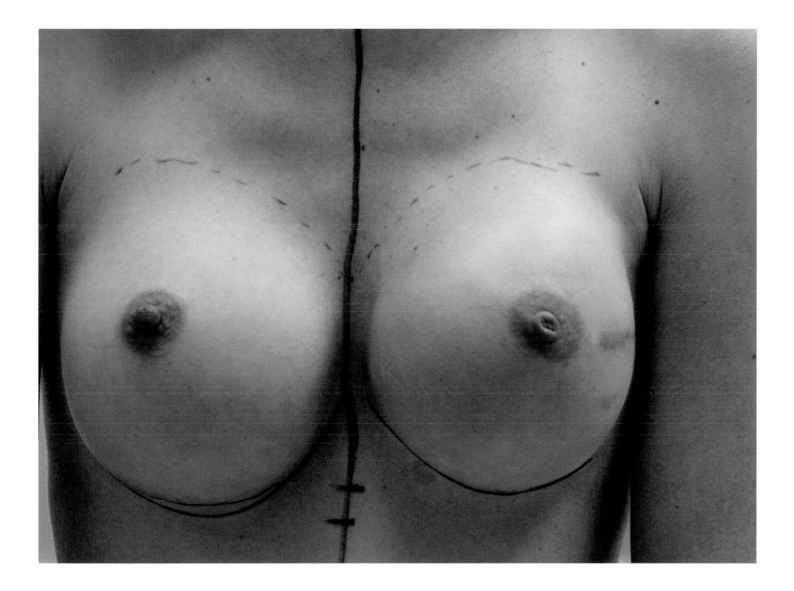

We have again made some markings on Shauna's chest. This will help guide us during this last surgery.

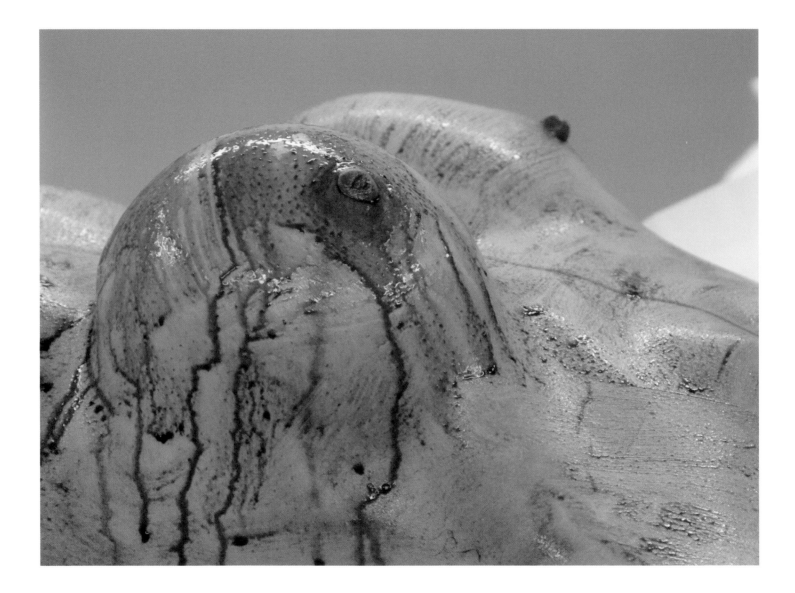

We have prepped the operative field with Betadine solution.

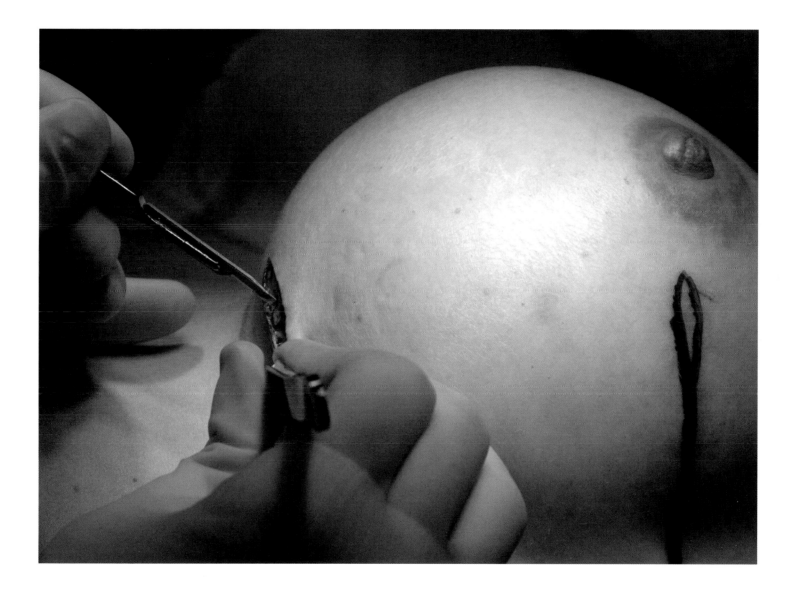

We start the surgery by revising a previous scar on the left breast.

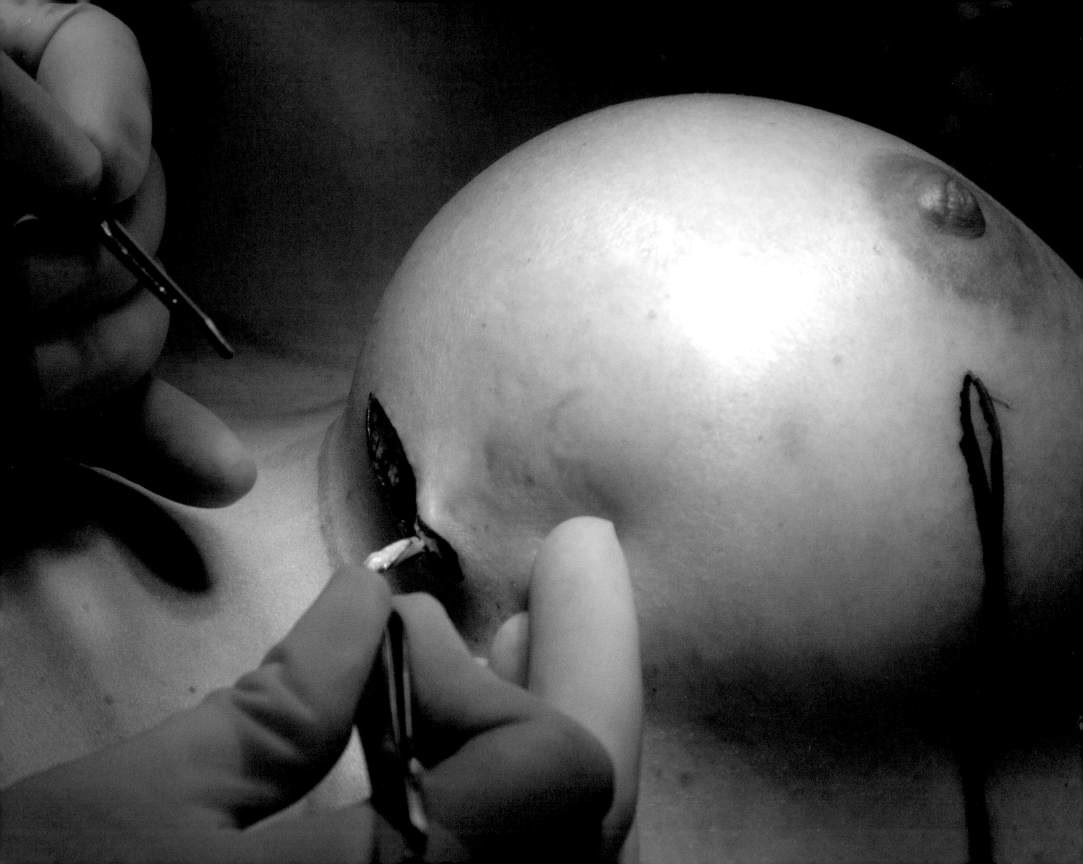

The mastectomy incision which will be used to remove the expander and insert the implant is marked in black (to the right of my right hand).

131

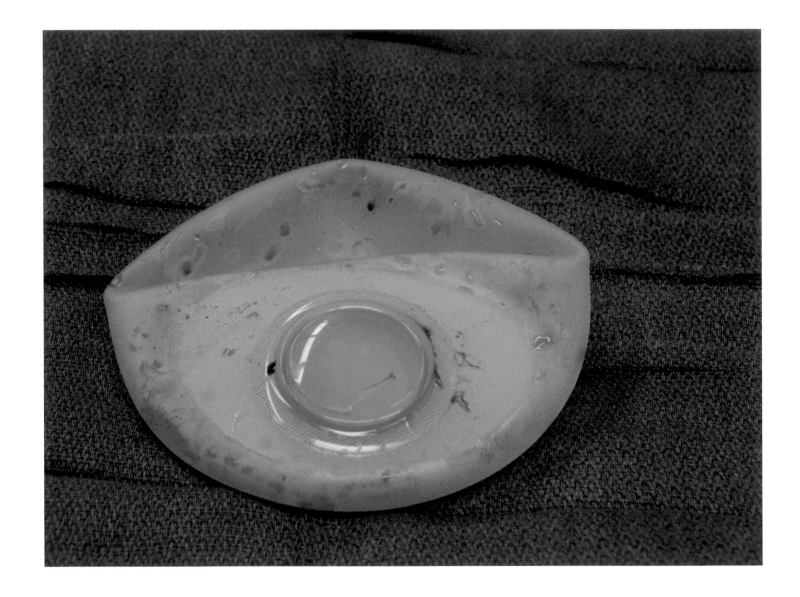

I deflate the expander and remove it from the left side.

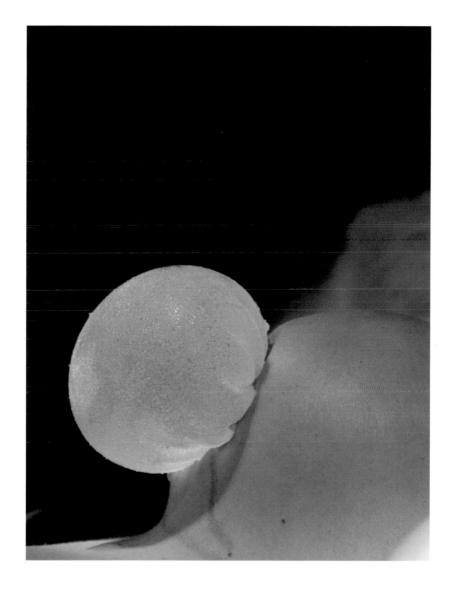

On the right side, we remove Shauna's old implant through an incision on the lower part of her breast.

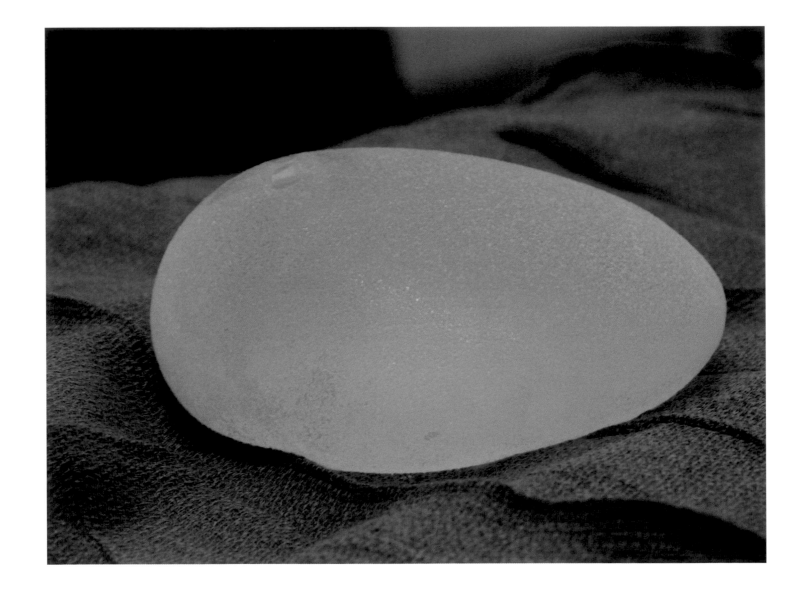

This is Shauna's old implant from her right breast.

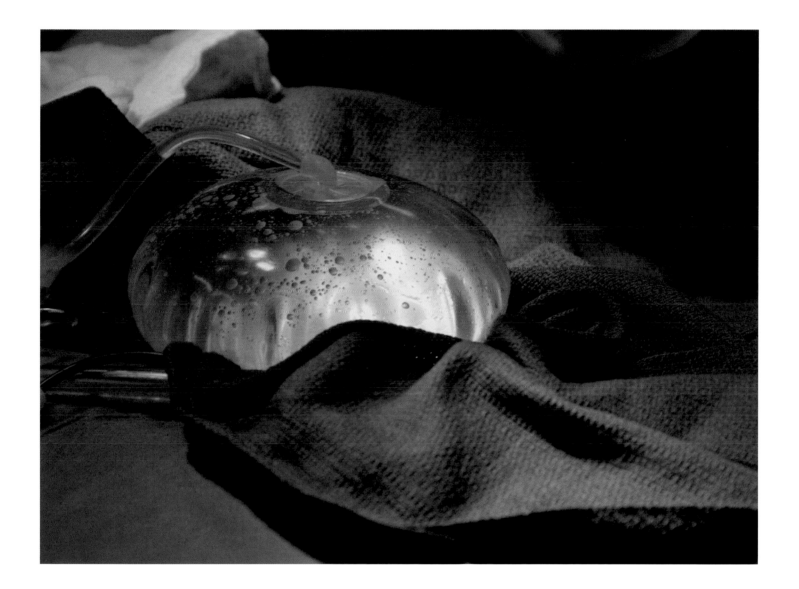

The next step is to place saline filled adjustable sizers into each breast pocket to try to figure out the best size and shape for symmetry.

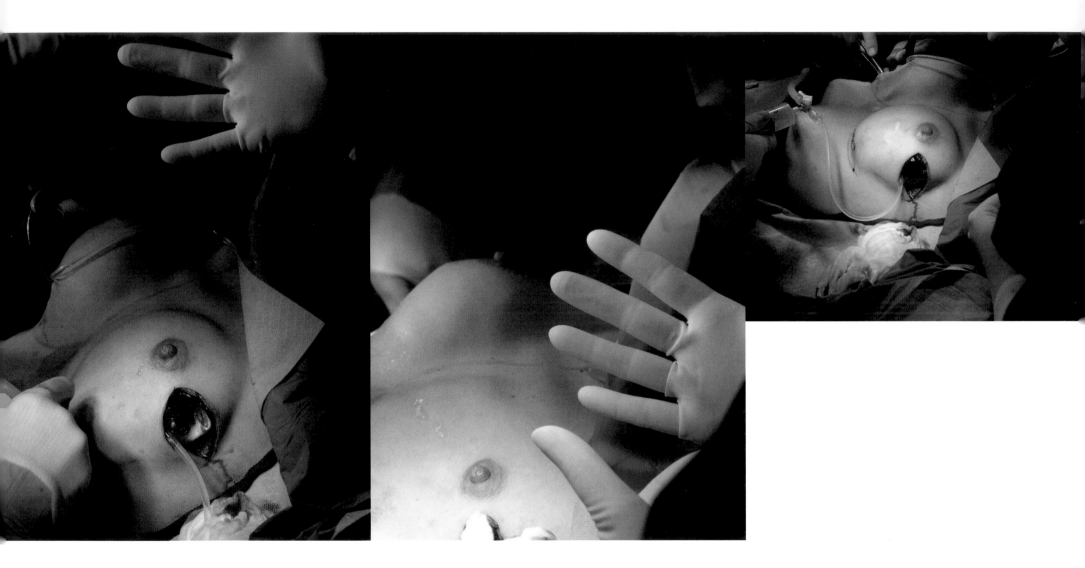

Here, we have sizers in both sides. We add fluid (saline) to each side to get the appropriate size.

The gloved hands in the photographs are helping us keep track of how much fluid we are instilling into each sizer.

137

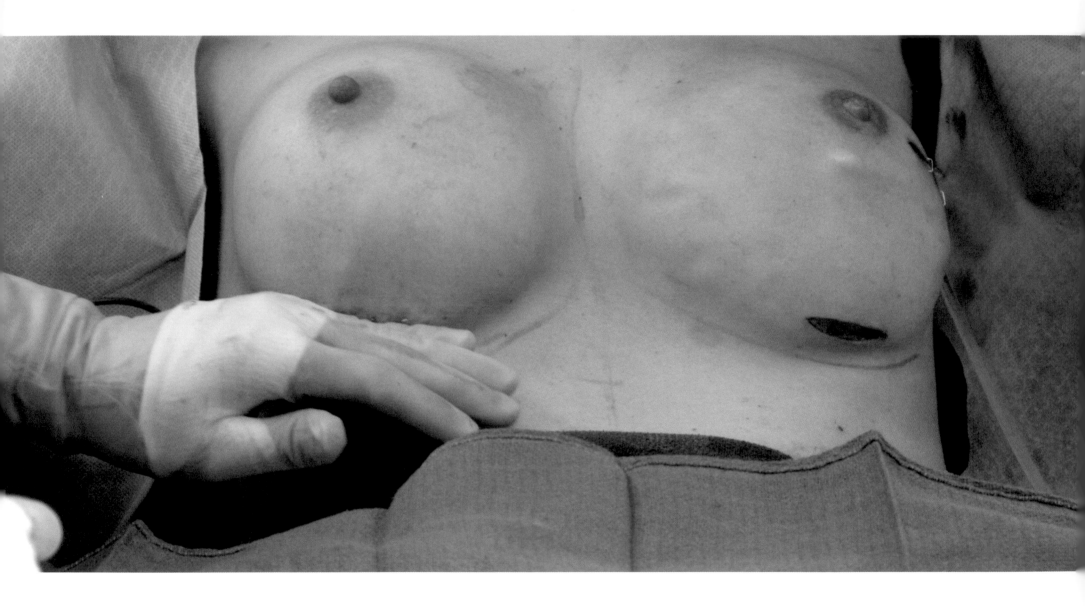

With the sizers in place we manually adjust the position of Shauna's breast so that it is in the best position.

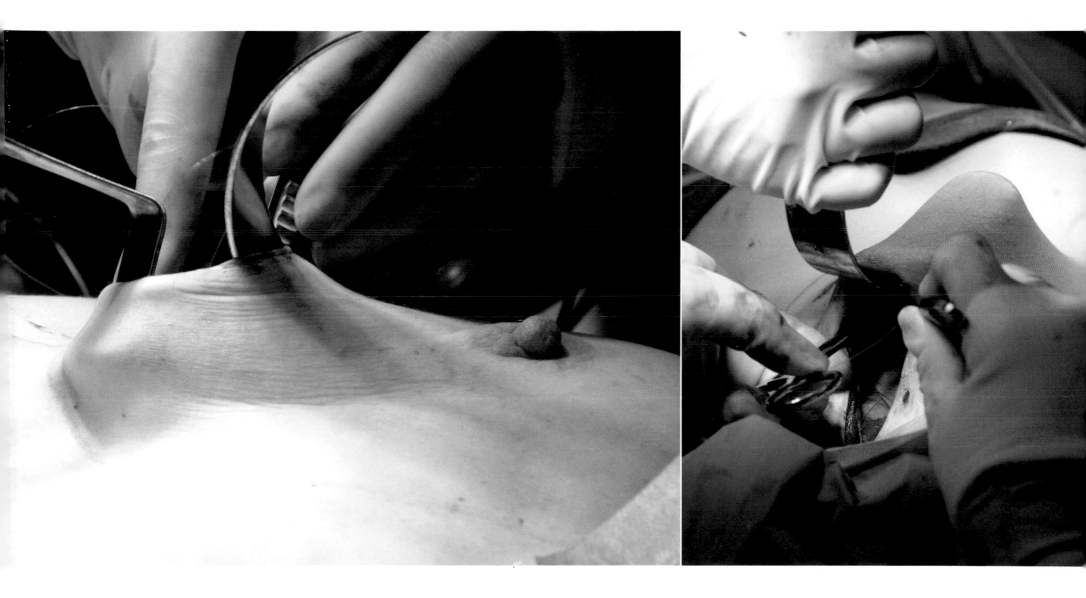

We remove the sizers and place sutures to define the new position of the breast.

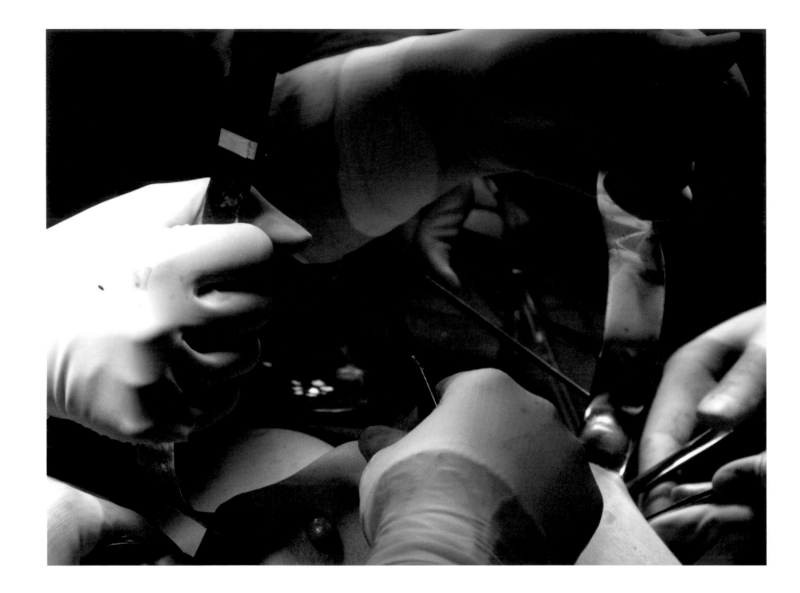

These operations require lots of hands.

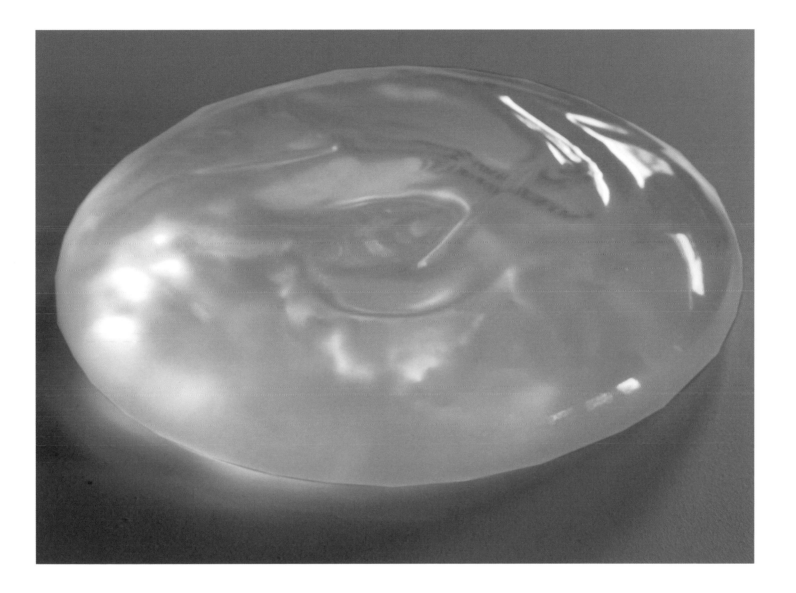

This is what Shauna's permanent implant looks like before it is inserted.

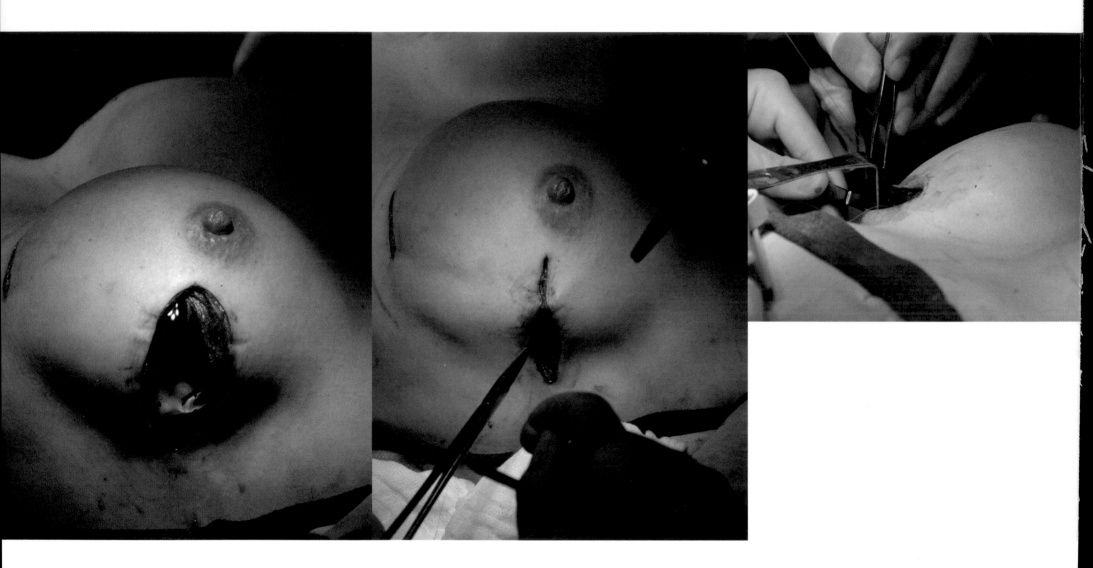

Once we have the implants in place, we again close the skin layer by layer.

(left) left breast   (center) left breast   (right) right breast

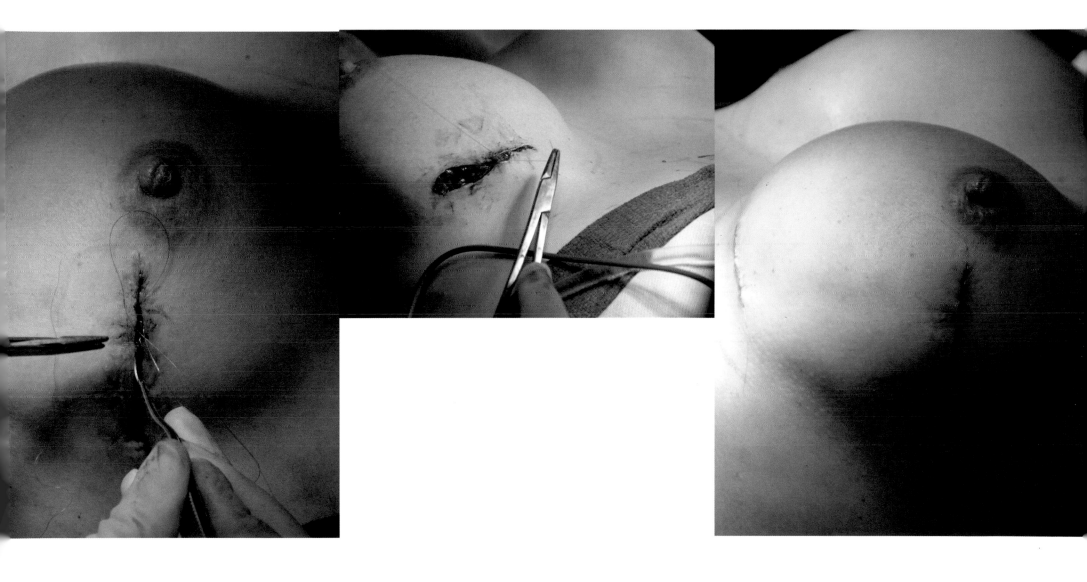

We use fine sutures in the skin.

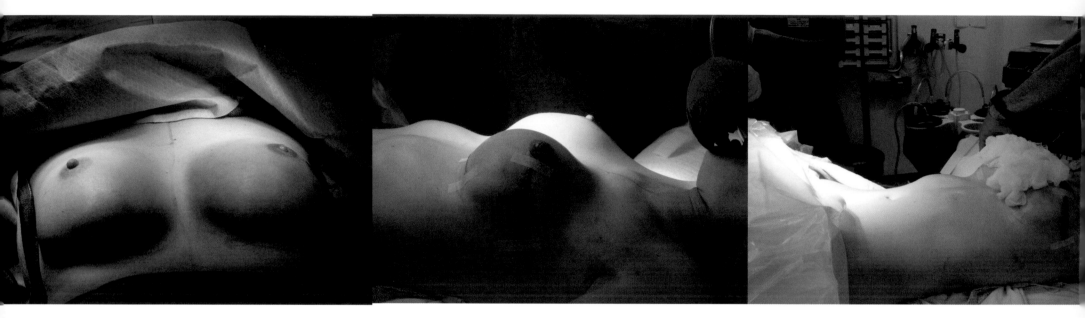

We apply the final dressings.

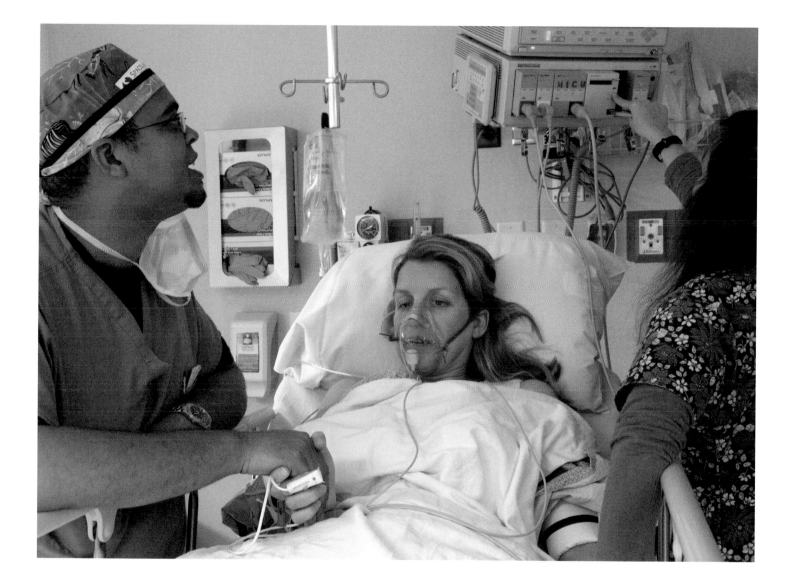

Shauna is awake and in the recovery room with her anesthesiologist by her side.

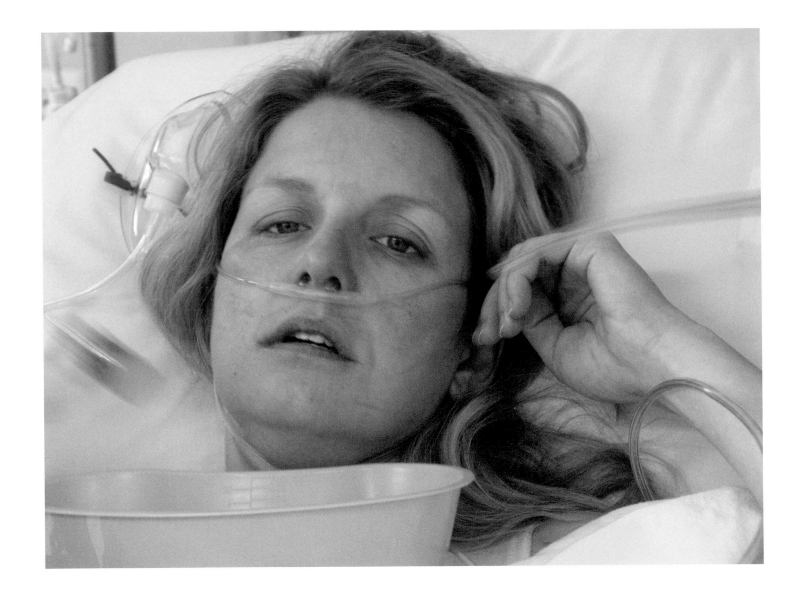

A wave of nausea can follow recovery from anesthesia.

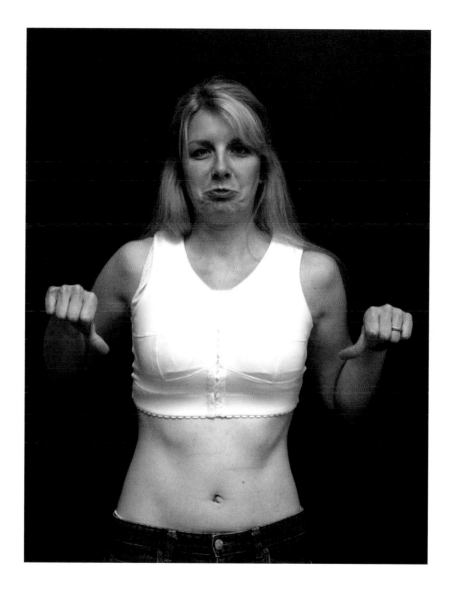

Shauna returns for her first post-op visit and is less than thrilled with the unflattering surgical bra.

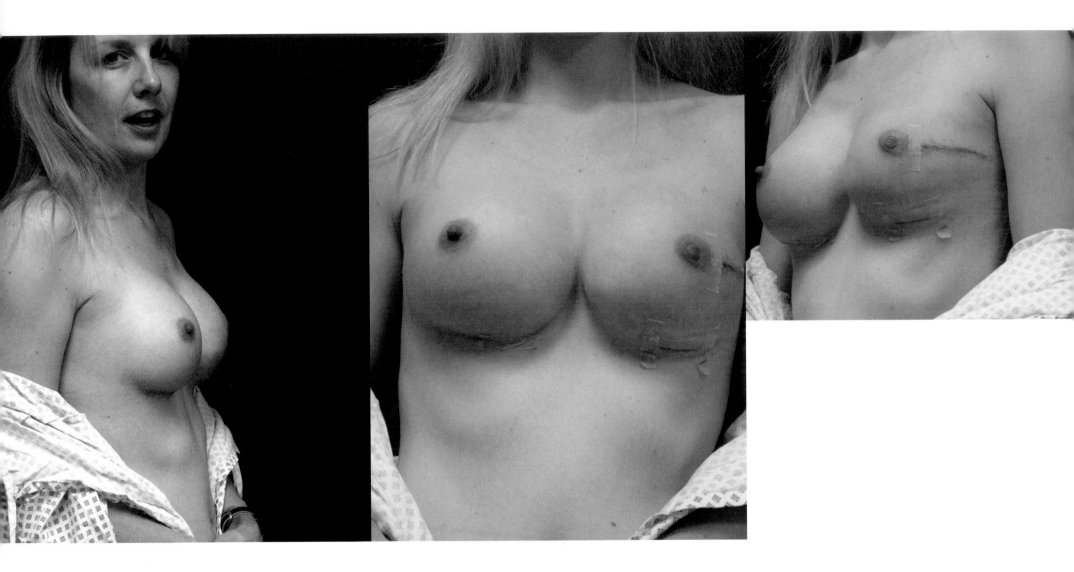

Shauna's incisions are healing well and the Steri Strip dressings are still in place. She has minimal bruising.

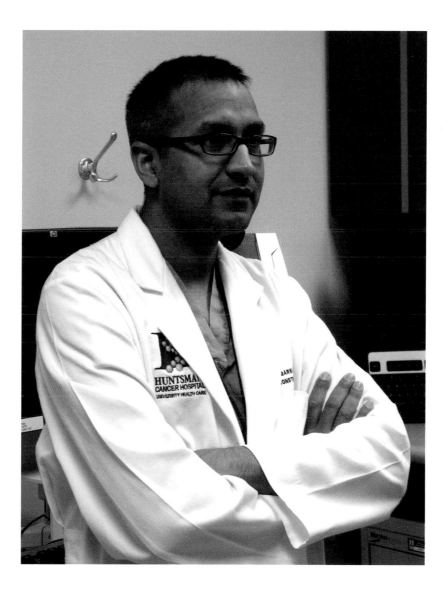

I discuss the previous surgery and tell Shauna that everything went well.

150

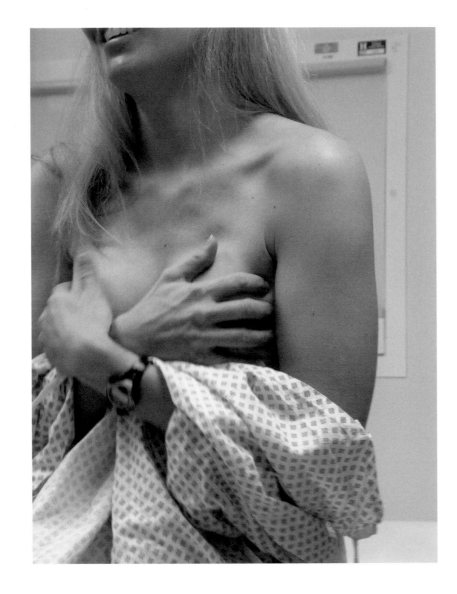

Despite having been examined numerous times previously, Shauna still has a little bit of shyness.

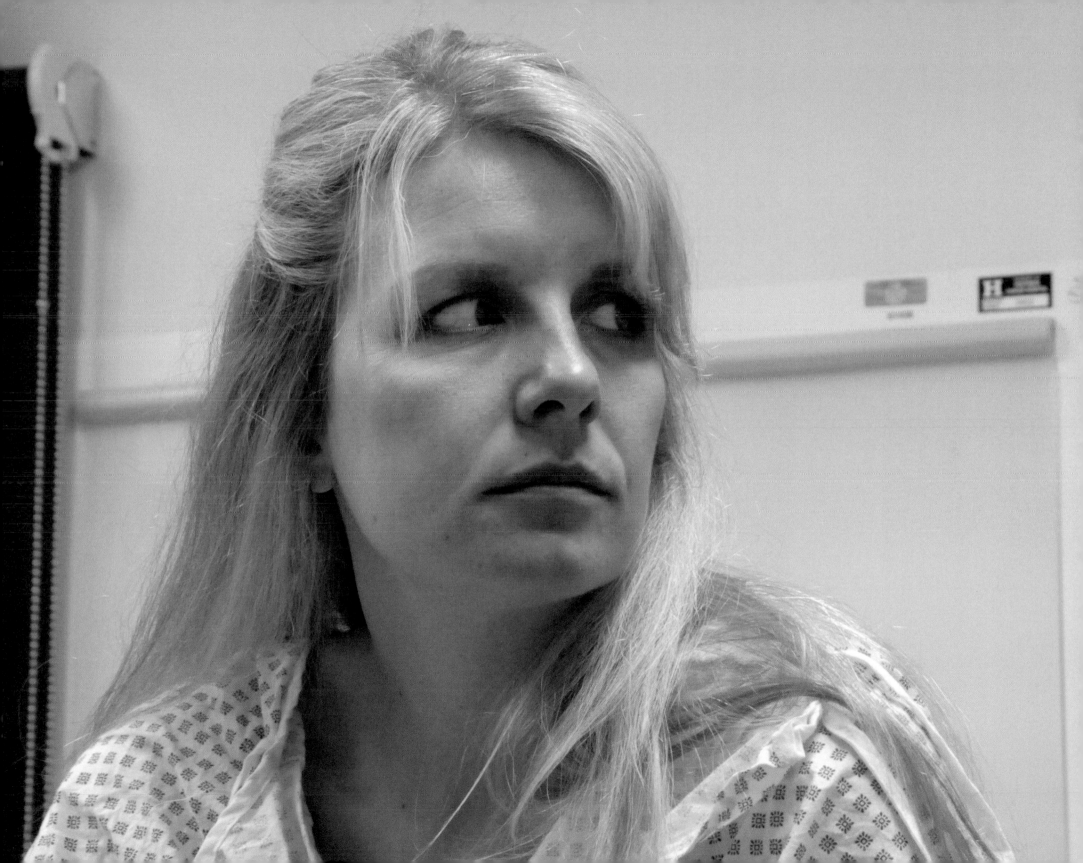

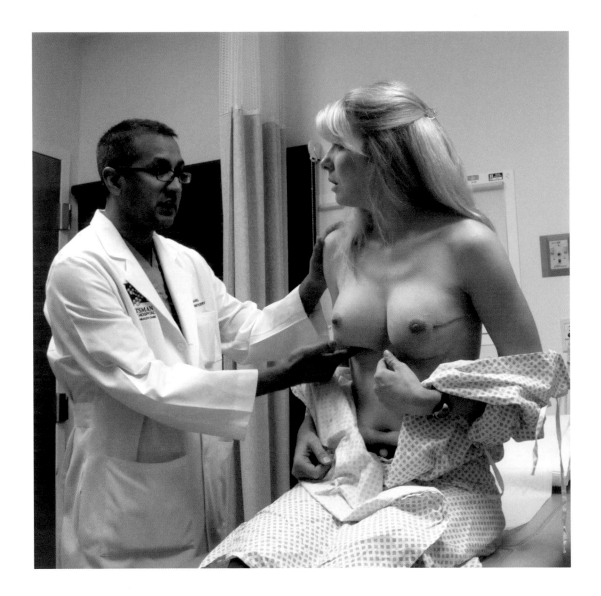

I explain to Shauna how the breast was raised by placing sutures on the underside.

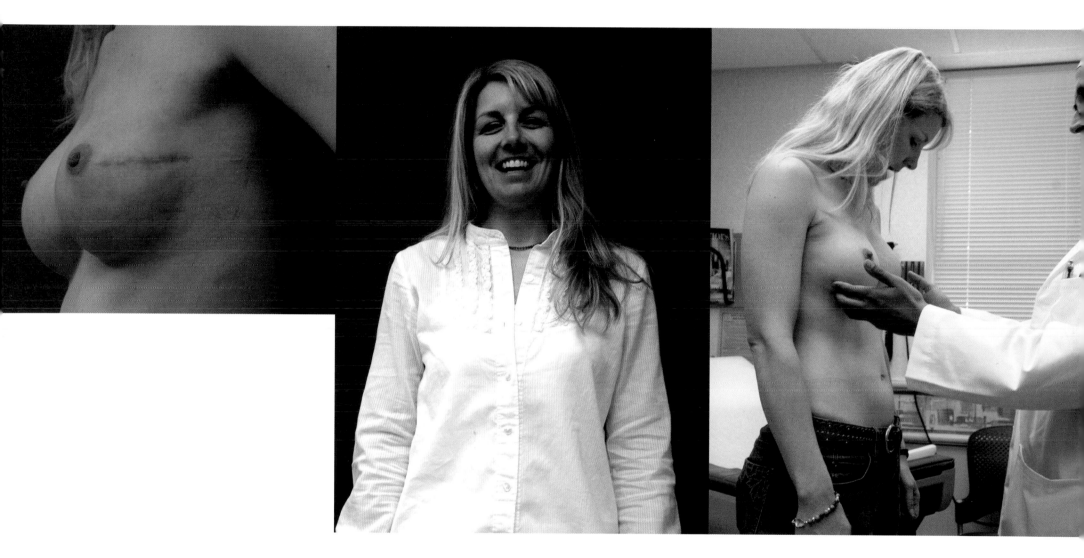

At the final clinic visit three months after the last surgery, Shauna is happy and has healed well.

Shauna: *I really like the idea of this procedure. What a great idea to slow the sagging of the breast. I will be perky for a long time!*

154

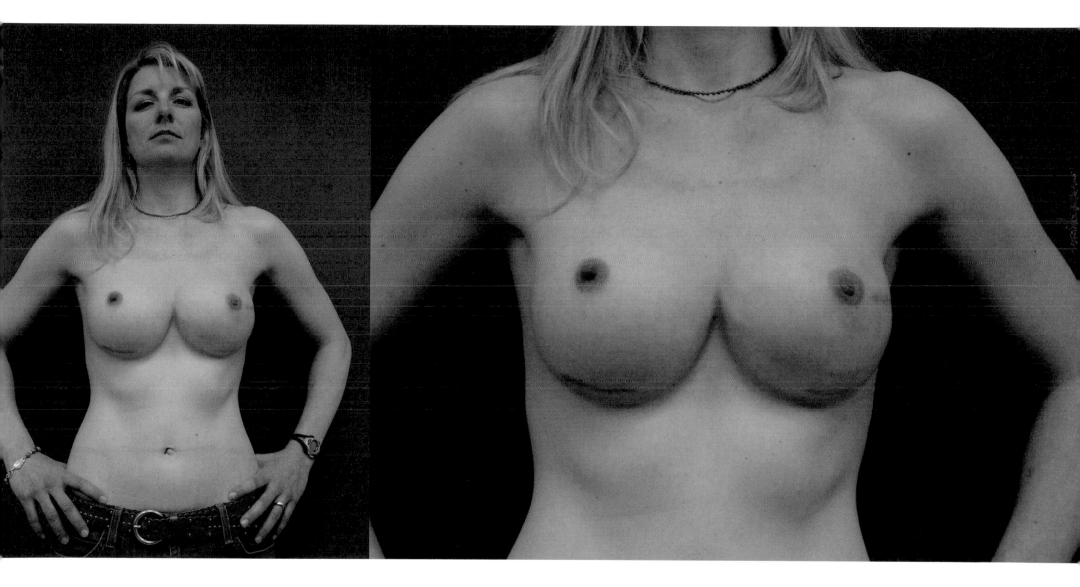

Shauna has good size and symmetry. Her scars are still red, but with time and massage they will begin to fade.

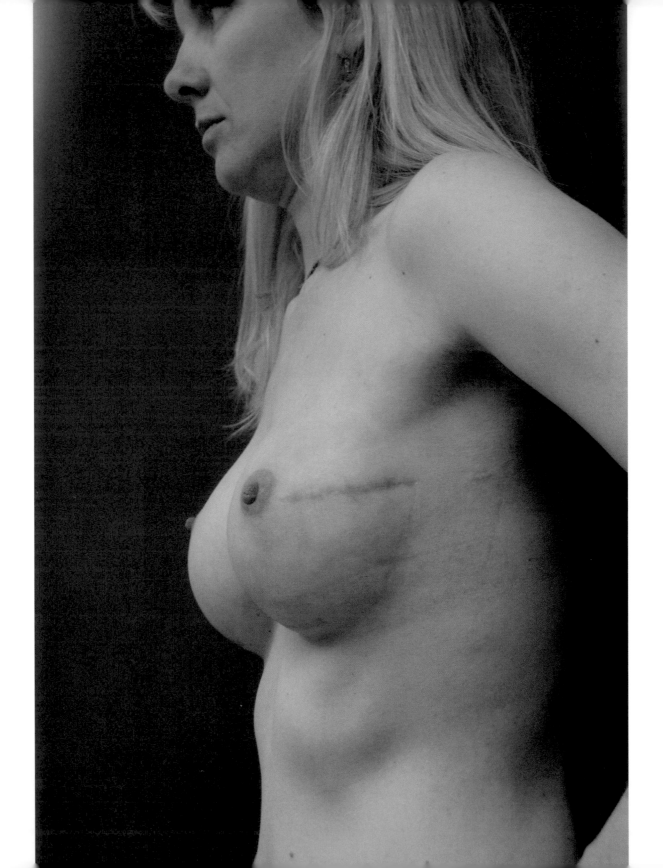

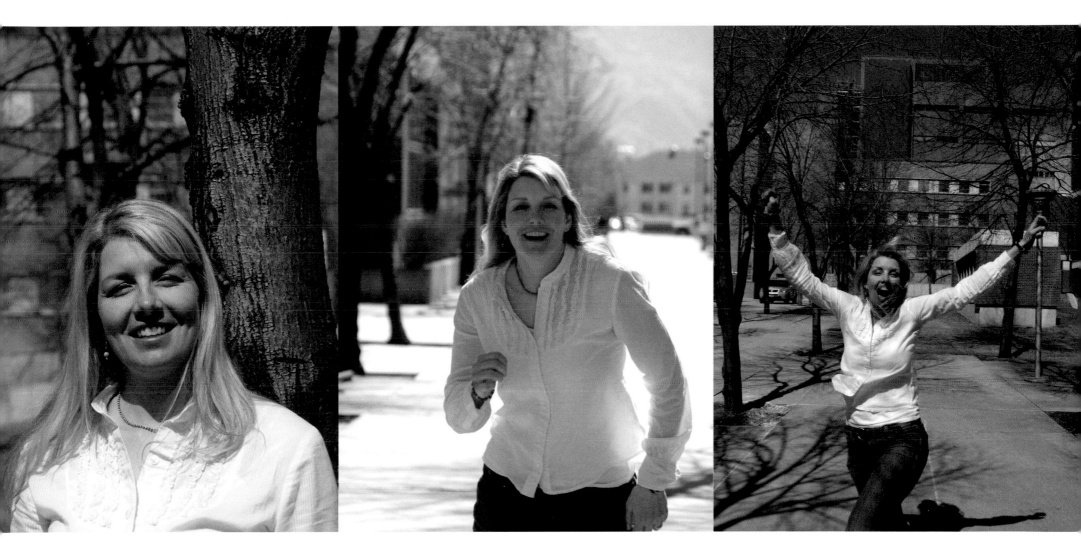

Shauna has been through a lot.

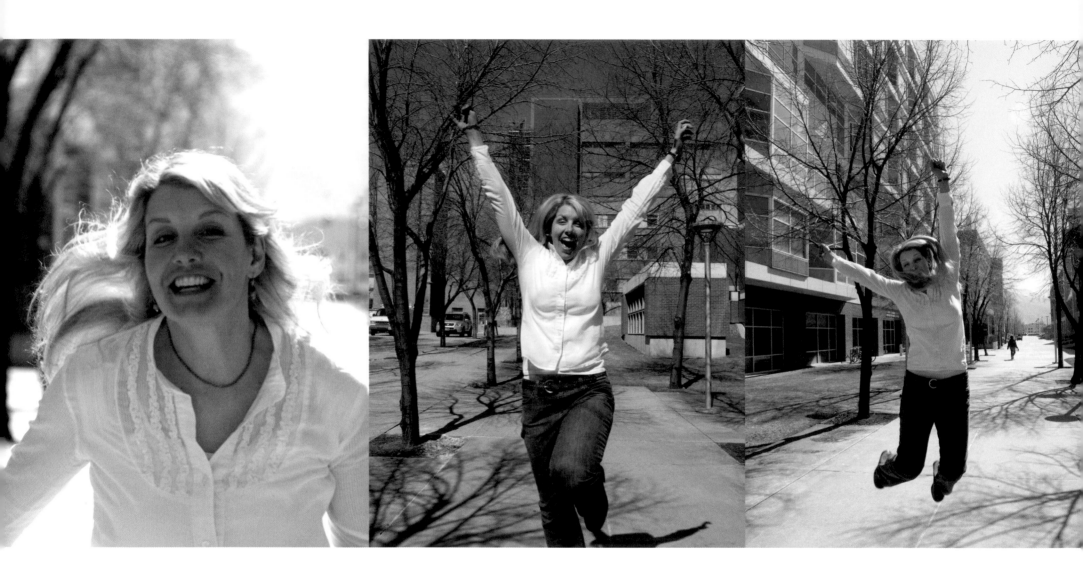

Now after two big surgeries and intervening expansions, she looks and feels like herself again.

Acknowledgements

We would all like to acknowledge the women in our lives (family, friends, and colleagues) who have struggled with breast cancer and the choices it forces on them and their loved ones. Thanks to the University of Utah and Huntsman Cancer Hospital, the Graduate Medical Education Office at the University of Utah Medical Center for moral support, and to the University of Utah School of Medicine Surgical Interest Group, which provided valuable feedback on an early draft.

We would like to thank Shauna Smith (superpatient!) for her strength and her willingness to share her experiences with other women, and for being willing to expose such a private part of herself to cameras and questions.

Dr. Neumayer: I would like to first and foremost acknowledge the support and encouragement from my husband, Dr. David Bull, as well as that from our children, Ashleigh, Andrew and AJ. My extended family, in particular my sister Patty, have all been supportive of this project as it has gone

159

from idea to reality. Also thanks to my brother-in-law and sister-in-law Donald Bull and Robin Berlin, who helped me with editing and connecting with other physician authors. In addition, this book would not have been possible without the great breast team at Huntsman (including Victoria and Vicki) and the great operating room staff. Lastly, to all my patients who amaze and encourage me with their bravery on a daily basis.

Dr. Agarwal: I would like to thank the wonderful women in my life: my wife Cori, my daughter Anjali, my mom Urmila, and my sisters Shobha and Jayshiri. Not only are they very supportive of what I do but they have all set great examples as strong women. Also, to my patients who are the bravest women I know.

Anne Vinsel: I would like to thank Kelly Johnson, for teaching me good OR manners, Marge Hansen, Cheri Peyton and TLC for getting me where I needed to be, Dr. SA for long distance encouragement and cheerleading, and Moose, always. Also thanks to my dog Spot, who had her cancer surgery the week before Shauna's and regained her happy dog smile. Don Kohan helped the project start and Alan Smith midwifed its successful delivery. Ken and Berkley at Pictureline and the geniuses at the Gateway Mac store contributed technical help when I was in way over my head. Breanna Stoll of the GME office gave thoughtful feedback on many versions. Any project like this depends heavily on people who gave freely

160

of their time when they didn't have to, like the patients' families who pilot tested early drafts, sometimes while waiting for their person to come out of surgery. I know one person's name, Karl Hurst-Wicker, an anesthesiology resident and friend of Shauna's who took the trouble to assign himself to Shauna's second surgery so he could keep her company in the recovery room. You others know who you are, even if we don't, and we are grateful for your help.

Finally, big thanks to Jeff Pollock, Penny Williams, Petra and Ricky Rose, Rusty and Karen Wales and others in the Salt Lake City Deaf community, who patiently kept repeating that a picture is better than a thousand words. I finally got it, guys!

Ravi Ahluwalia: I would like to thank my family, who each contributed in their own unique way to making me the person I am today. As things change, they have been a constant. I'd also like to thank anyone who ever took the time to teach me or guide me in the right direction. And Anne Vinsel; were it not for her vision this book could not have happened.

All of us would like to thank Kitty Grigsby for doing our prepress, Cindy Maher and Bruce Bracken for guiding us through the publishing process, and the color wizards at Worzalla for their beautiful printing job.

161

162

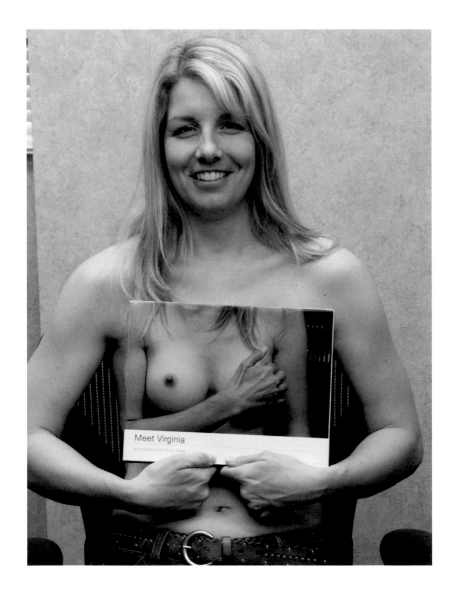

Meet Virginia!

Technical Notes

These photographs were taken using available light.

Cameras used were a Nikon D300 with an AF-s micro Nikkor 105 mm lens (vibration reduction) and a Nikon D70 with an aspherical Nikon .56m-1.9 ft zoom lens.

The high quality jpeg and tiff images were edited on a MacBook Pro and an iMac using iPhoto, and the original book layout was created using iBook.

Glossary

American Society of Plastic Surgeons: www.plasticsurgery.org

anesthesia for breast cancer surgeries: Most mastectomies and reconstruction surgeries are done under general anesthesia with the patient fully asleep.

anesthesiologist: This is a medical doctor who ensures that the patient is asleep and pain free during surgery. He/she also ensures that the patient's vital functions (breathing, circulation, etc) are functioning properly during the operation.

attachments: strings of tissue that attach one structure to another

autoimmune disease: a group of diseases in which the immune cells of one's body react against the body. Examples of such diseases are lupus, rheumatoid arthritis, and scleroderma.

axilla, axillary tissue: armpit, tissue in the armpit

Betadine: a brownish orange colored antiseptic

breast cancer:
    invasive: (large size is larger than about 2 inches/5 cm): Cancer
        cells have pushed through the walls of the ducts or lobules

    pre-invasive (also called ductal carcinoma in situ, or DCIS): Cancer
        cells haven't pushed through the walls of the ducts

    inflammatory: cancer is present in the skin lymph channels. This
        usually results in the breast being red and the look of fluid
        collecting in the skin (sometimes called "orange peel"
        because the skin can look dimpled like the peel of an orange)

    locally advanced: lots of disease in the breast and armpit,
        sometimes growing through the skin

    close margins: the cancer is within a millimeter/.04 inches of where
        the surgeon cut to remove the breast tissue

breast implant (permanent): This is a balloon-like implantable device used
to reconstruct the breast. It can be filled with saline or silicone.

breast reconstruction, immediate: Immediate breast reconstruction refers to the placement of a tissue expander, implant, or the body's own tissue during the same surgery as the mastectomy.

cadaver skin, human: This is donor tissue (skin) from humans which is used to help create the pocket in which the expander is placed. This tissue has been processed to remove the cells with the tough connective tissue proteins remaining. Over time, this tissue becomes incorporated into the patient's body.

capsular contracture: This is the process of scar hardening which can occur after placement of a breast implant. When implants are used for breast reconstruction, capsular contracture rates can be higher than when implants are used for cosmetic breast enhancement. It can result in an unsatisfactory aesthetic result.

cauterization: use of electrocautery to stop bleeding or cut through tissue

chemotherapy (chemo): medicine used to kill tumor cells

clavicles: collar bones

CO2: A gas called carbon dioxide. CO2 is what cells in the body make as they use energy. If your CO2 is too high, it means you aren't breathing rapidly enough; if it is too low, you are breathing too quickly.

cosmetic augmentation: This is the process of enhancing the shape and size of the breast using breast implants.

dermis: deep layer of the skin

dissection: Dissecting is cutting down through flesh in an organized way to reach the tumor or area that needs to be removed; also removing the tumor or breast.

dressings: bandages

ducts: tubes leading from the breast tissue to the nipple

drainage tubes: tubes placed in and around the reconstructed breast to help drain fluid (plasma and blood) that may accumulate after surgery.

electrocautery: a multipurpose surgical tool that lets surgeons cut through skin and flesh, and also burn closed tiny blood vessels that would otherwise seep and create blood in the wound. It works a lot like a woodburning tool.

expander, tissue expander: This is basically an adjustable water balloon that has a valve where fluid can be added after the surgery. We start with it not all the way filled so we don't have problems with the blood supply of the overlying skin, then over the course of weeks or months, add more water/saline in clinic.

fascia: a tough layer, usually found on top of or separating muscle from other tissue.

forceps: A surgical instrument that looks like long tweezers, used much like chop sticks to pick up tissue. In fact, they are often called "pick ups."

Geiger counter: an instrument that measures radiation, used to track injected radiolabeled material during sentinel lymph node dissection. It consists of two parts, a probe and a counter. The probe touches the patient's body, and the counter figures out how radioactive that location is.

grade (of tumor): how the cells look under the microscope. The grade is an indicator of how well behaved the tumor cells look (Grade 1--like teenagers left home alone for only a short time period) or not so well behaved (Grade 3--like teenagers left for a weekend with no adult supervision) or somewhere in between (Grade 2—you get the picture).

her-2-neu receptor: Docking station found on the cell wall of this specific type of cancer. We have a drug that specifically acts on this receptor (Trastuzimab—herceptin) that we can use for patients whose cancer cells have this receptor.

hormone receptors: Docking stations found on the cell wall for hormones (progesterone and estrogen). If the cancer cells are found to have these, the hormones dock in these stations and stimulate the cells to grow. If these are found on the cancer cells, we have several ways to treat these cancer cells, either by blocking the receptor, or by keeping the patient from making the hormone.

hot spot—where the radioactivity is the strongest. This is where the surgeon will look for the sentinel lymph node(s) to remove.

imaging: pictures, usually some type of xray, mammogram, ultrasound or MRI

implant:
    temporary: usually a tissue expander

    permanent: This is the final breast prosthesis and can be either
        saline or silicone.

induction: the start of anesthesia (going to sleep for surgery)

inferior, inferiorly: towards the feet or down

inframammary fold: the crease under the breast

lateral: side

local recurrence: cancer coming back in the breast, skin or on the chest wall

lumpectomy: taking out a lump. Specifically for the breast it means removing part of the breast, usually referring to the area of the tumor with a rim of normal tissue.

lymph nodes: glands found throughout the body that work as filters to catch bacteria and other debris. Negative lymph nodes means that no cancer cells are detectable in the lymph nodes that have been removed (a good thing). Positive lymph nodes means that cancer cells have been found in the lymph nodes that were removed and examined by a pathologist. This could be an indication that the cancer is more extensive than we would hope or that it is spreading to other areas of the body.

   axillary lymph node dissection: taking out lymph nodes from the
      armpit
   sentinel lymph node biopsy: a technique that allows the surgeon to
      identify and remove the first node(s) that an area drains to.

massage: Scar massage is the process of rubbing scars to help them soften and fade.

mastectomy:
    total skin sparing (nipple sparing mastectomy): removal of all the
        breast tissue but leaving the entire skin envelope (including
        skin of nipple and areola

    skin sparing: removal of all the breast tissue, and a very small
        island of skin, i.e. only the skin of the nipple and areola. The
        incision is made in a circle around the outside of the areola.

    traditional: removal of all the breast tissue with an island of skin (the
        island is centered around the nipple and areola, so this part of
        the skin is also removed. This island is usually shaped in an
        oval with points on either end (also called an ellipse).

medial, medially: toward the center

nipple areolar complex: the confluence of the ducts as they head up
through the nipple (the tissue right under the skin of the nipple and areola)

nuclear medicine: a specialty of medicine that uses radioactively labeled
materials to assist doctors

oncology, oncologic: relating to cancer

operative field: the part of the patient's body where the surgery will take place. Everything else is draped with sterile cloths and paper coverings; only the operative field is exposed to the scalpel.

orientation suture(s), marking suture(s)—stitches that tell the pathologist which way the tissue was originally lined up in the patient's body. It serves the same function as "this way up" arrows on a package.

oxygen saturation: the percentage of red blood cells that are carrying oxygen

palpation: feeling, touching

pectoralis major muscle: the name of the biggest muscle found underneath the breast

peritumoral technique for injecting radiolabeled dye: injecting (with a needle) the dye fluid around the tumor

planes: natural separations between types of tissue (e. g., skin and breast, muscle and fat)

post op: the time period after a surgery

quadrant: Surgeons divide the breast into four equal quarters, so that they can easily talk about location.

radiation therapy: high dose radiation delivered to specific areas to treat cancer

radiolabeled material/radioactive tracer: material that has a bit of radioactivity attached to it

reconstructive surgery: operations to recreate what had to be removed because of cancer or other disease

retractor: a tool used in the operating room to hold tissue out of the way

revising (previous scar): Revising a scar is surgery performed to remove an unsightly scar and replace it with a less prominent scar.

saline: salt water

silicone: Silicone is a man-made polymer of elemental silicon and oxygen. It has many uses as a rubber, sealant, and for medical devices. It is used in the production of breast implants due to its gel-like consistency and biologic inertness.

sizers, adjustable: These are balloon-like bags that are sometime used in the operating room to help the surgeon decide which final size breast implant to choose.

skin envelope: the skin covering the breast

skin flaps: the skin that used to cover the breast but that now covers the chest or the reconstruction

skin hooks: tools used in surgery that hold the edges of the skin without squeezing it

174

staged (surgical) approach: surgery that requires more than one procedure. Breast reconstruction is often staged and can include different surgeries for tissue expander placement, definitive breast reconstruction (with either implants or the patient's own tissue), and contouring.

Steri Strip: tape-like bandages

sternum: breast bone

subareolar (technique, injecting radiolabeled dye): injection of dye into the tissue of the breast underneath the nipple/areola

subcutaneous (tissue): usually fat

surgical field: where we are performing the operation. Usually it has been cleaned with antiseptic solution and marked around the edges with sterile towels so nobody gets confused.

suture: stitch; suture is the material, sometimes looks like thick thread, other times looks like fishing line. Unlike fabric sewing where the stitches are connected, most surgical stitching is done one stitch at a time, and each stitch gets its own knot.

tissue expander/skin expander: see expander above

traction, counter traction: pulling the tissue one way and the other to help with the operation

Frequently Asked Questions
about breast cancer surgery

Q: How much do the different parts of the process hurt?
A: Typically, the first surgery hurts more than the second surgery, mostly because the pectoralis muscle is traumatized and feels like a bad, bad Charlie horse.

Q: What about working after the surgeries? Using your arms? Lifting/holding young kids?
A: After the first surgery most people require 3 weeks off work and off from heavy lifting. After the second surgery, most people resume their routine in 5-7 days.

176

Q: How long will it take to recover completely?
A: This depends on many factors, including age, physical condition before surgery, whether you have had radiation or chemo, etc. And some people just heal faster than others.

Q: Will my insurance cover the surgery?
A: Yes, including surgery for the unaffected breast to achieve symmetry. Of course, there may be co-pays and you may have to pay a percentage, depending on your insurance.

Q: After I am healed, what will sensation be like?
A: There is usually no nipple sensation and some breast sensation.

Q: I've heard about lymphedema, which can apparently be quite physically limiting.
A: Lymphedema may result from lymph node removal or radiation.   It is swelling, which can be quite severe, in the arm/armpit area. It is not shown or discussed in this book because Shauna did not experience it.